To Dr. Randy

For your support
in making a
difference and
changing lives.

RB

Image Guided Dermatologic Treatments

Robert L. Bard

Editor

Image Guided Dermatologic Treatments

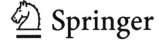 Springer

Editor
Robert L. Bard
The AngioFoundation
New York, NY
USA

ISBN 978-3-030-29234-8   ISBN 978-3-030-29236-2   (eBook)
https://doi.org/10.1007/978-3-030-29236-2

This Springer imprint is published by the registered company Springer Nature Switzerland AG
The registered company address is: Gewerbestrasse 11, 6330 Cham, Switzerland

To my wife, Loreto, whose vision made this work reality

Dermatologic Foreword

Image-guided dermatologic treatments present the latest clinical options in digital skin imaging, optical/laser systems and advanced immunologic therapies. The targeted approach adds onto recent publications of the International Dermal Ultrasound Group comprehensively cataloging diagnostic features of benign and malignant dermal disorders. This book is written for clinicians in medical and allied fields where dermatologic diagnosis with the least invasive option is required. It is organized so that the text advances from the dermatologic sciences to advanced imaging and radiologic breakthroughs, thus serving as a reference guide for the dermatologic community to assist clinical diagnosis with the new sonographic, CT, MRI and nuclear medicine procedures now refined for dermatologic and subcutaneous pathologies.

Initial chapters on benign and inflammatory diseases are precursors to advanced treatises on pigmented lesion analysis and hidradenitis suppurativa. The chapter on melanoma skin cancer and malignant melanoma is followed by updated concepts of melanoma treatment including genetic markers and the use of PET/CT to ensure continued therapeutic success.

Subspecialty chapters on dermal trauma from foreign bodies and burns to iatrogenic scar formation provide an explanation with regard to wound healing and cicatrix treatment using OCT and microlaser technologies. Filler materials and aesthetic treatment complications are highlighted, including the possibility of irreversible blindness currently occurring worldwide. The unique biomechanical features of the foot and ankle unit merit discussion of the weight-bearing effects on the skin and subcutaneous tissues as well as the lethality of acral melanoma.

State-of-the art reflectance confocal microscopy now diagnoses cancers with near-histologic accuracy and is used during real-time Mohs micrographic surgery to guide border excision potentially converting the usual multistage operation into a one-step procedure. Cellular imaging resolution quantifies inflammatory processes such as psoriasis and lupus erythematosus both by characteristic anatomic appearance and quantitative physiologic capillary blood flow in the clinically noted hyperemic areas. Moreover, optical computed tomography delineates basal cell cancers and noninvasively verifies postoperative tumour margins sparing patients further biopsy. It has also successfully guided treatment of melanoma within the tissue perfusion parameters restricted to this modality. Hyperspectral imaging is promising although a recent study demonstrated a 36% specificity in cutaneous melanoma detection. Proteomic mass spectroscopy, Raman spectroscopy and genetic expression profiles are still in clinical development, thereby elevating high-resolution Doppler sonography as the new "gold standard" for noninvasive skin cancer examination.

A final note is the importance of vessel density quantitative perfusion imaging in the analysis of cancer biology with application to verify successful therapies. Similarly, inflammatory disorder treatments may be quickly assessed using tissue neovascularity as a complementary surrogate marker with visual clinical assessment. Treatment decisions may be adjusted in a timely manner if vascular imaging criteria indicate suboptimal clinical response. The great clinical success of biologics linked to an increased incidence of lymphoma may be noninvasively confirmed or ruled out by real-time 3D ultrasound Doppler exam of subcutaneous growths or cutaneous manifestations occurring during therapy.

The contributors are dermatologists trained in ultrasound diagnosis and proceed to chapters authored by interventional radiologists, dermatopathologists and specialists in advanced optical and microscopic dermatologic analysis that provides a comprehensive reference for noninvasive diagnosis techniques and image-guided minimally invasive treatment options.

Using image guidance, treatment decisions may be adjusted in a timely manner if vascular criteria indicate suboptimal clinical response, and new lesions may be noninvasively confirmed or ruled out by real time 3D ultrasound Doppler exam of subcutaneous growths or cutaneous manifestations occurring during therapy. This textbook advances the application of new imaging technologies by dermatologists and assists radiologists to focus on the distinctive clinical aspects of skin and allied subcutaneous disorders.

Lebwohl Mt Sinai Hospital, New York, USA   Mark Lebwohl

Radiologic Foreword

Although diagnostic ultrasound technology originated in the USA for military and industrial purposes, regulatory mandates restricted development in certain medical fields. In 1973 Dr. Bard trained at the Danish Medical Center where the previous student became the Director of Ultrasound at Harvard Medical School. Thus, he was aware of the significance of alternative European imaging protocols that are not fully recognized in the USA. At the 1st International Symposium on Melanoma (1990) at the Mount Sinai Medical Center, one of the presenters noted that X-ray or CT scan has no role in the diagnosis of cutaneous melanoma. Following that presentation, as a speaker and one trained in high-resolution breast, ophthalmic and dermal ultrasonography, Dr. Bard visibly rebutted the previous claim and showed sonograms of the skin produced by the Bronson Ophthalmic 10 MHz unit, demonstrating the capability to image both cutaneous and uveal melanoma. Since then, advances in ultrasound transducer design and allied optical imaging technologies allowed accurate depth determination of skin cancer and real-time assessment of surgical margins and onsite detection of malignant regional lymphadenopathy.

In October 2001, Dr. Bard participated in the Journees Francaises de Radiologie in Paris, a major conference in Europe attended by 18,000 radiologists, and witnessed the potential of three-dimensional (3D) technology for multiplanar imaging of the soft tissues and Doppler vascular mapping of the blood vessels of the skin, nail and subcutaneous regions. Although the equipment was approved for use all over the world, including the USA, there was not one unit that was used in North America for dermal investigation. As of this writing, Dr. Bard is one of the few physicians using the Volumetric 3D ultrasound in the USA for advanced cancer imaging. Physicians now use ultrasound routinely for diagnosing breast cysts or visualizing gallstones. Ultrasound is excellent for guiding needles to aspirate fluid or inject within a joint. Urologists rely on sonograms for prostate biopsy, and anaesthesiologists perform nerve blocks under sonographic control. The medical community has not yet embraced the advanced technology that offers 3D imaging similar to an MRI that shows the location of the tumour and if it has spread. Moreover, it simultaneously measures intratumoral cancer aggression. Internists and family physicians refer patients with skin problems to dermatologists. Radiologists do not see patients for this type of exam because patients are not sent for skin imaging by local practitioners, in large part because this is a relatively new diagnostic modality for them and the current FDA regulations limit advanced applications.

This book has been written to enlighten physicians, nurses, health providers and patients into the leading edge of medical diagnosis and the latest therapeutic options using image-guided treatments. Medicine without compassion for the patient may not be worth dispensing. It is very easy today to cure diseases and destroy the human being in the process, as witnessed in radical surgeries, chemotherapies and immunotherapies. This book aims at preserving human dignity and personal choice while simultaneously controlling cancer. His purpose in writing this book is threefold, that is to:

- Provide practical knowledge of the specific disease
- Offer hope and cure based on proven scientific research
- Encourage realistic empowerment for medical challenges

Advances in functional imaging, such as Doppler flow probes and nuclear medicine combining PET/CT and MRI protocols, have provided the possibility of image-guided treatment for cutaneous and metastatic skin cancers and soft tissue sarcomas measure treatment effect of the immunologic and oncologic tools we use now. The new noninvasive optical technologies of reflectance confocal microscopy and optical coherence tomography are refining diagnosis and creating options for image-guided treatment.

Today's health-conscious society with instant access to the Internet means that physicians have to answer specific questions from educated patients regarding the latest diagnostic modalities and minimally invasive treatment options. For example, adults seeking reassurance about pigmented lesions and children with suspicion of melanotic malignancies may instead need treatment for forgotten splinters, thorns, glass and other foreign bodies that may be subdermal in location and, thus, invisible to the spatially restricted human eye and impalpable to latex-gloved fingers. Ultrasound accurately noninvasively detects and performs in the office setting accurately and rapidly due to the high resolution and low cost of today's sonographic equipment. Our duty is to keep ourselves up to date about the importance of ultrasound diagnosis and provide this knowledge and opportunity to the enquiring sophisticated patient.

Major changes in the incidence, diagnosis and treatment of skin cancer and benign dermal/subdermal diseases highlight a singular need for an up-to-date source of diagnosis and minimally invasive therapy of dermal and subcutaneous tumours. Melanoma cancer occurs at a median age of 28 years, and the incidence is increasing rapidly. This suggests that patients in their 30s are developing cancer that may be missed by the current screening technologies such as dermoscopy, confocal microscopy and near-infrared optical devices. Delays in treatment due to misdiagnosis have led to lawsuits. The earlier the detection of tumours, smaller lesions are discovered, and focal nonsurgical treatments become realistic options for standard operative modalities with potential long-term postoperative side effects. Inflammatory lesions, such as acne vulgaris and hidradenitis suppurativa, with a 52% recurrence rate, often extend beyond the optically limited clinical exam. Recognition of subdermal fistulae or pseudocysts in the deeper tissues may dictate suspension of topical treatment and alter systemic management.

Currently the ageing population is pursuing cosmetic procedures and anti-ageing protocols towards a youthful look in increasing numbers. Image guidance allows physicians to measure skin thickness and depth of fat tissue as well as evaluate the elasticity of the skin and subcutaneous tissues improving thermal and electromagnetic treatment outcomes. Medical imaging maps the arteries, veins and nerves providing preoperative landmarks reducing postoperative bleeding and avoiding nerve damage. Irreversible blindness has been documented worldwide following injection of fillers and fat transfer implantation. Imaging permits safer therapeutics with increased effectiveness and decreased treatment times. Image-guided treatment by nonsurgical or minimally invasive modalities greatly reduces patient anxiety and the possibility of postoperative disfigurement. Minimally aggressive tumours may be treated medically and followed by interval scans or destroyed by focal thermal ablation. Biopsies of certain abnormalities may be averted or postponed.

Benign disease and cosmetic treatment options are further improved by 3D image reconstruction and 4D volumetric mapping of regional anatomic structures. This rapidly acquired data set allows for accurate serial comparison in follow-up exams and speeds up surgical therapies, since the adjacent nerves and arteries are pre-mapped and visually displayed. The ability to follow the course of nerves allows for ultrasound-guided nerve block anaesthesia and decreases the possibility of nerve injury during treatment. Image-guided hydrodissection techniques strip away irritated or entrapped nerves from inflamed tissues reducing pain and increasing muscle functionality in a short office visit. New cryoprobes target nerves of the face producing muscle relaxation, such as Botox injections, without the cost and bruising sequelae. Breast, buttock and facial implants may be periodically assessed to determine migration and avoid complications, such as fat and skin necrosis. Noninvasive imaging identifies subdermal fillers or implants as to content and location that present as dermal disorders due to poor patient history and material migration over short or very long time periods. Translocation of fillers and movement of implants with vascular compromise or nerve entrapment may be observed and release therapies instituted with real-time verification of success.

Dermal sonography has been used since 1980 and complements other modalities, such as dermoscopy, reflective confocal microscopy, optical coherence tomography, dermal CT and MRI scanning, that together diagnose, stage and grade cancer. It evaluates the extent of certain benign disorders such that biopsy may be limited or avoided. This has been useful in following the side effects of injected fillers which may occlude arteries or implants that migrate causing pressure necrosis. Additionally, an aesthetic physician faced with a potentially poor history of prior surgical encounters benefits by screening the anatomic field to avoid needling subcutaneous calcifications or injecting into forgotten silicone deposits and displaced implants.

Diagnostic Applications

Clinical diagnosis of nonmelanoma skin cancer (NMSC) is generally accurate; however, the depth of a tumour is unknown. Imaging alerts the surgeon whether the surgery will be limited to a single excision or extensive requiring skin graft or cartilage replacement. Clinical diagnosis of malignant melanoma is 54% accurate by histology and 20% accurate by non-microscopic clinical modalities. Many benign pigmented lesions are removed preventively. There is one malignant melanoma found per 33,000 nevi. Ultrasound screening of pigmented lesions is highly accurate and well tolerated. MRI studies are currently sensitive but not specific or practical for screening. Dermoscopy and other optical technologies have increased in clinical acceptance and application and are currently performed as complementary exams to dermal sonography. Pathologists now preview clinical pictures of a suspected lesion before they finalize the readings due to the inherent variability of interpretation. The finding of a subclinical metastatic focus near the lesion provided by the newer ultrasound and optical technologies facilitates histologic interpretation. Optimal aesthetic treatments require advanced knowledge of the size, volume and depth from the skin surface. The preoperative determination of the presence of fat, vessels, high dermal melanin content or cystic fluid collections allows better choice of the energy source and optimizes treatment parameters. For example, acne lesions in the upper epidermis respond best to blue light, while deeper epidermal lesions fare better with red light. Solar lentigines and freckles are situated in the upper epidermis, whereas melasma and Becker's nevi are located in the lower epidermis.

Ultrahigh-frequency units with 50 micron resolution of the epidermal barrier may support newer nutritional approaches to optimal healing, skin quality and appearance and enhance related biological systems. Therapeutic progress is substantiated by epidermal changes during treatment, which assures the patient and aesthetic team that the treatment is successful. For example, recent studies have supported the use of probiotics to improve skin health due to their effects on immune function and inflammation, as well as oxidative stress, glycaemic control and tissue lipid content. Antioxidants, selected for function and their ability to support multiple biological systems, are targeted to protect cell membranes and to restore elasticity and function. This enhances the cell's uptake and utilization of essential nutrition. Botanicals provide effective protection from UV exposure that causes significant damage via lipid peroxidation in skin cells. Melanin may be protected by targeted and properly balanced dietary nutrition and supported with topical treatments. Improved skin cell turnover and optimal hydration can also be achieved through nutritional interventions using compound formulations. This approach combines dietary intervention, targeted nutrition and an understanding of key nutritional ingredients for cosmeceutical supplementation offering a dietary plan and nutritional protocol for long-term skin health and healing modified for patient use.

Image-Guided Biopsy and Treatment

New computer programs use nanotechnology, artificial intelligence and cybernetic modalities for accurate image-guided biopsy and treatment options. Employing 3D sonography with Doppler, the physician manually or robotically targets the area of highest tumour neovascularity. This is critical since only part of a mass may be cancerous and the malignant tissue may be missed on nontargeted punch or shave biopsies. The application of alternative imaging technologies with ultrasound permits image-guided biopsies that spare the adjacent neurovascular bundles. Immediate cytologic confirmation of tumour cells permits the withdrawal of the biopsy needle and insertion of a laser fibre, focused ultrasound device or cryogenic probe immediately treating the proven tumour. Thermocoupled sensors prevent overheating of the adjacent nerves and sensitive tissues. Following ablation, the zone of destruction is confirmed with Doppler, contrast ultrasound or other vascular imaging techniques. Inflammatory lesions that are deeply seated may be approached by stereotactic image-guided subdermal injections or targeted biopsies if necessary. This outpatient procedure allows the patient to return to work immediately. RF thermoprobes with temperature auto cutoffs prevent thermal skin damage as does image-guided subdermal saline standoff injections. Similar user-friendly and cost-effective modalities may replace other therapies in the near future. At the 2019 ASLMS (American Society of Lasers in Medicine and Surgery) meeting, cutaneous melanoma with in-transit metastases was reported to be successively treated by laser technologies.

Future Developments in Cancer Angiogenesis

Angiogenesis in the normal physiologic state is a new vessel formation in the areas of cellular reproduction, vessel development and wound healing. Proangiogenic and antiangiogenic factors are balanced to control these functions. Pathologic angiogenesis is the abnormal proliferation of blood vessels presumed to be stimulated by central hypoxia within the tumour. While vascular endothelial growth factor (VEGF) is the most important factor in the development of immature tumour vessels, it is not suitable as a clinical measurement in skin cancers.

Advances in ultrasound imaging include very high-frequency probes, from 22 to 100 MHz, providing image resolution of up to 30 microns and ultrasound contrast agents allowing real-time imaging of tumour neovascularity. The technical aspects of Doppler flow detection with subharmonic imaging of microbubbles are discussed in other articles. Histopathology demonstrated that tumours not only vary markedly over their surface volume in appearance but also have variations in microvasculature directly proportional to invasive aggression and metastatic potential. Studies using tumour immunohistochemical markers show strong correlation with tumour neovascularity with subharmonic contrast ultrasound. 3D ultrasound imaging quantifies pathologic vessel density in different quadrants of the tumour permitting more accurate biopsy targeting. Contrast bubble imaging, not yet FDA-approved for the skin, will shortly add a new dimension in the assessment of treatment by quantitative changes in tumour vessel density measurement.

Summary

Portable high-resolution sonography units are now available in offices. It distinguishes midline critical vascular lesions, such as sinus pericranii, from nonvascular masses. Tumour depth accurately assessed shortens Mohs treatments. Cartilage invasion and aberrant nerves or arteries may be assessed preoperatively. Subcutaneous masses, such as cysts or foreign bodies, are quickly diagnosed. Increased use of biologics with the potential side effect of lymphoma means a patient with an unexpected subdermal mass can have certainty that it is indeed a benign lipoma or simple cyst readily differentiated from a metastatic node or lymphocytic cancer. The more dermatologists and plastic surgeons use the imaging capacities of sonography and allied radiologic cutaneous imaging, the more they will find its attributes essential to the modern practice of skin disorder therapies.

Catalano Italian Cancer Institute, Naples, Italy   Orlando Catalano

Acknowledgements

Chris Renna
Richard Menashe
Jesse Stoff
Mark Lebwohl
Hooman Khorasani
Mona Darwish
Manu Jain
Gary Goldenberg
David Goldberg
Andrew Rossi
Bruce Katz
Robert Schwarcz
John Melnick
Emil Toma
Staff
Maryann Sta. Rita
Aimee Arceo
Members of FDNY
Jim Hayhurst
Salvatore Mirra Jr.
John Signorile
Richard Marrone
Chief Bob Checco
Jimmy Amman
Sal Banchitta
Cancer Foundations Organizers
Cheri Ambrose
Peggy Miller
Bret Miller
Debra Black
Lori Nash
Ginny Salerno
Kristie Moore -
9/11 Memorial Museum
Alice Greenwald -President & CEO • Director
Anthony Gardner
Jan Seidler Ramirez

Contents

Advantages of Sonography of Benign Skin Diseases

Claudia Patricia González Díaz

1.1 Introduction

Ultrasound has become a very important diagnostic modality in the investigation of dermatological diseases [1–3], since it allows early diagnosis, determines the degree of activity and severity of the disease, and provides accurate anatomical information optimizing preoperative planning for surgical procedures. Although magnetic resonance is frequently recommended for pre-surgical assessment, it requires the use of intravenous contrast and has been shown to be less effective in the detection of lesions smaller than 3 mm [4]. While other diagnostic modalities like optical imaging technologies have important limitations to assess the depth of the lesions, ultrasound is a noninvasive diagnostic method, without ionizing radiation, suitable for the diagnosis and monitoring of multiple benign dermatological pathologies.

1.2 Technical Considerations

The study must use a high-resolution multichannel linear transducer from 15 to 22 MHz, which clearly defines surface structures such as skin layers and delimits lesions up to 1 mm in thickness or performs deeper exploration of subcutaneous or muscular lesions that can simulate injuries of superficial origin [5, 6]. It is essential to have a trained radiologist with precise knowledge of normal dermatological anatomy and pathology. Sonographic tools should be used as an expanded field of vision that allow us to scan the totality of the lesion and involvement of adjacent structures, Doppler for assessment of the vascular pattern in real time and 3D reconstruction [7, 8] for better anatomic mapping.

1.3 Normal Skin

It is constituted by three layers: epidermis, dermis, and subcutaneous cellular tissue [9].

The epidermis has a highly pleomorphic cellular content and is not vascularized; its nutrition is carried out by diffusion of the dermal circulation. The main cell types of the epidermis are keratinocytes, melanocytes, and Langerhans cells [10, 11]. Ultrasonography observes a highly hyperechoic linear layer due to its high content of keratin and collagen.

The dermis corresponds to the supporting structure of the skin; histologically it is dominated by organized collagen packages and provides the mechanical function of the skin. It includes vessels, lymphatics, nerves, the deep portion of the hair follicles, and sweat glands. In ultrasound it

C. P. G. Díaz (✉)
MSK, Bogotá, Colombia

Instituto Diagnostico Medico Idime, Bogotá, Colombia

© Springer Nature Switzerland AG 2020
R. L. Bard (ed.), *Image Guided Dermatologic Treatments*,
https://doi.org/10.1007/978-3-030-29236-2_1

is visualized as a hyperechoic band of variable thickness depending on the area of the body. In elderly people or those with high solar exposure, it can become hypoechoic due to trophic changes [12]. The subcutaneous cellular tissue is constituted by fatty lobes separated by septae ultrasonically appearing as a hypoechoic layer, separated by hyperechoic linear septum (Fig. 1.1).

1.4 Benign Tumors

This category includes, among others, epidermal cyst, pilomatrixomas, lipomatous tumors, pilonidal cyst, scarring endometriosis, and dermoid cyst.

Epidermal cysts are caused by the implantation of epidermal elements in the dermis and subcutaneous cellular tissue and in the infundibular portion of the hair follicle. Ultrasound shows a mass with oval, hypoechoic configuration with a duct that connects it to the surface called the punctum, and posterior acoustic reinforcement is noted (Fig. 1.2). The "onion" pattern has also been described in ultrasound by the curvilinear arrangement of keratin. Giant cysts present a "pseudotestis" pattern [13], because it is very similar to the normal ultrasound aspect of a tes-

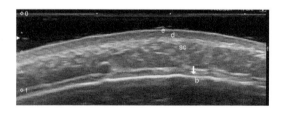

Fig. 1.1 Aspect of the normal skin of frontal region, e, hyperechoic epidermis; d, dermis; sc, subcutaneous cellular tissue. Arrow, frontal muscle; b, cortical frontal bone

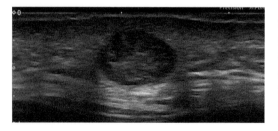

Fig. 1.2 Typical image of an epidermic cyst, oval, well-defined image with posterior acoustic reinforcement

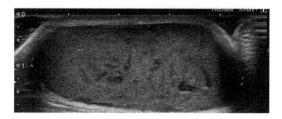

Fig. 1.3 Giant epidermal cyst with pseudotestis configuration

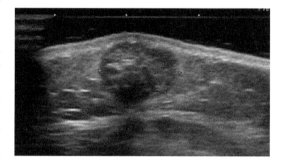

Fig. 1.4 Typical aspect of pilomatrixoma with multiple calcification pattern with posterior acoustic shadow in some of the calcifications

tis (Fig. 1.3). Pilomatrixomas are benign tumors derived from the hair matrix [14]. They are more common in children and young adults, especially affecting the head, hand, neck, and limbs [15]. The clinical diagnosis may be incorrect in up to 56% of cases as they can easily be confused with other benign tumors, such as epidermal cysts [16]. The classic sonographic appearance is that of a "target" lesion characterized by a solid hyperechoic mass with a hypoechoic halo, punctiform calcifications with posterior acoustic shadow as a diagnostic key, which can be single or multiple [17]. In the periphery, it may present some degree of vascularization (Fig. 1.4).

Lipomas are the most frequent soft tissue tumors and are derived from mature fatty tissue and can be single or multiple [18]. They are called superficial when they are located in the subcutaneous cellular tissue and deep when they are below the fascial/muscular plane. They are called typical when their content is exclusively fatty. They may have associated mesenchymal tissue and connective or capillary tissue and be named fibrolipomas or angiolipomas according to the predominant tis-

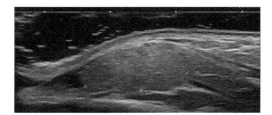

Fig. 1.5 Typical lipoma: oval mass, homogeneous texture, hyperechoic with defined contours, located on the upper eyelid

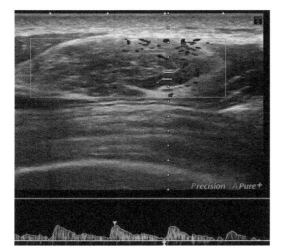

Fig. 1.6 Mass of heterogeneous texture, predominantly hyperechoic with linear tracts and discrete vascularization in the periphery; the pathology reported angiolipoma

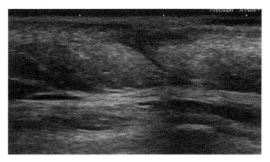

Fig. 1.7 Typical ultrasound image in the inter-gluteal region corresponding to pilonidal cyst

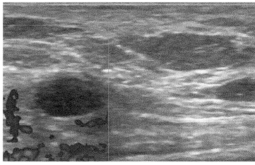

Fig. 1.8 Patient with a history of cesarean section, with mass in subcutaneous cellular tissue on the cicatricial path, with vascularization at Doppler examination; the pathology confirmed scarring endometriosis

sue component. Atypical lipomas are the ones that have potential malignant transformation such as liposarcomas. The typical lipomas in ultrasound appear as oval masses markedly hyperechoic that follow the transverse axis of the skin layers, when their sonographic presentation is characteristic and the diagnostic certainty is very high [19–22] (Fig. 1.5). Atypical lipomas in ultrasound are solid masses, with predominantly hyperechoic heterogeneous texture with hyperechoic tracts, and their edges may be well or poorly defined. Angiolipomas show some degree of vascularization at Doppler examination (Fig. 1.6).

Pilonidal cyst is the most common lesion of the inter-gluteal region. They are composed of a pseudo-cystic structure that contains a network of hair and keratin [23]. In ultrasound they are seen as hypoechoic sinuous collections with internal echoes, which occupy the dermis and subcutaneous cellular tissue [24] (Fig. 1.7).

Scarring endometriosis is the implantation of endometriosis tissue in postsurgical scars of cesarean sections or gynecological surgeries situated in the layers of the skin or subcutaneous cellular tissue. Although infrequent, it is a cause of pelvic pain. The most frequent cause is the implantation of cells of the endometrial tissue at the time of surgery. The characteristic ultrasound presentation is that of a solid, hypoechoic mass in the postoperative path area, with a detectable flow in the Doppler scan [25] (Fig. 1.8).

Dermoid cysts are masses that contain remnants of skin tissue such as keratin, hair, and stratified epithelium with a thick capsule that originate along the embryonic closure lines [26]. They are usually seen in the upper outer quadrant of the orbit in children and young adults. Other areas of less frequent localization are midline off the neck,

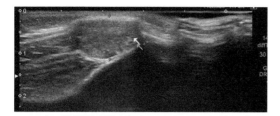

Fig. 1.9 Patient of 3 months of age with subdermal mass, in external quadrant of the orbit with typical presentation of dermoid

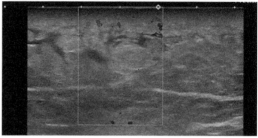

Fig. 1.10 Patient with cellulitis in the abdominal wall; bundles of hypoechoic fluid dissect the subcutaneous cellular tissue, and there is increased vascularization on Doppler examination

nasal, forehead, mastoid area, and torso [27–29]. Ultrasound observes a round anechoic mass, well delimited with a thick capsule (Fig. 1.9). There should not be calcifications or vascularization since the absence of bone or cartilage is what differentiates a dermoid from cystic teratomas [30].

Congenital vascular disorders have been covered in recent textbooks, and these malformations are developmental abnormalities and do not constitute vascular tumors. Suffice it to mention that Doppler vessel imaging is important both for diagnosis and follow-up of treatment efficacy.

1.5 Infectious and Inflammatory Processes of Skin

Infectious includes superficial and deep cellulite, abscesses, and chronic inflammatory processes such as hidradenitis suppurativa and psoriasis.

Cellulitis is an acute inflammatory condition of the skin that is characterized by pain, erythema, and heat in the affected area [31]. It is usually caused after a bacterial infection from *Staphylococcus aureus* and pyogenic *Staphylococcus*. Even when the diagnosis is clinical, ultrasound is used to differentiate between superficial and deep cellulitis. In superficial cellulitis, the infectious process involves epidermis, dermis, and subcutaneous cellular tissue without extending to the muscular fascia. Ultrasound shows an increase in the thickness and echogenicity of the three layers of the skin, hypoechoic liquid in the septae, and increased neovascularization at Doppler exploration (Fig. 1.10). In the other hand deep cellulitis, is the extension of the inflamatory process to deep tissues, such as muscular fascia or muscles, and

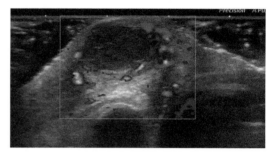

Fig. 1.11 Pre-septal abscess in a teenager patient; ultrasound shows a hypoechoic collection with some echoes inside it and with increased flow in the periphery, at Doppler examination

it is denominated as fasciitis or myositis with or without necrosis depending on the affected area. Necrosis is observed as irregularly defined cystic areas with increased vascularization at Doppler examination.

Abscesses correspond to the presence of infection and pus in a liquid collection. The most frequent etiological agent is *Staphylococcus aureus* [32]. Among the common causes of organized collections are hematomas, ruptured epidermal cysts, and inflamed pilonidal cysts. Cellulitis and abscesses are the first cause of hospitalization of drug addicts [33]. Abscesses can be organized or not. In ultrasound, unorganized abscesses are observed as hypo- and hyperechoic, irregular collections with variable degree of vascularization in the periphery [34] (Fig. 1.11). Organized abscesses show defined hypoechoic collection with a peripheral pseudocapsule. There may be hyperechoic points with "comet tail" artifacts corresponding to air

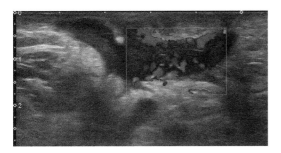

Fig. 1.12 Subdermal fistulous hypoechoic tract in a patient with hidradenitis suppurativa with marked inflammatory activity demonstrated by increased vascularization inside the fistula

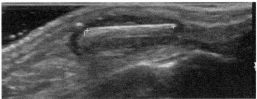

Fig. 1.13 Patient with foot trauma, 2 months later, presents soft tissue mass; ultrasound confirms the presence of hyperechoic linear image corresponding to foreign body-type wood chip and hypoechogenicity in the periphery by the formation of granuloma

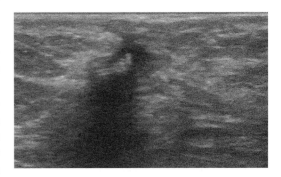

Fig. 1.14 Patient with postoperative scar mass; the ultrasound shows a typical image of granuloma, with irregularly marked hypoechoic nodule with hyperechoic center

inside. Drainage guided by ultrasound is very useful both to define the etiological agent and to perform definitive treatment thereof [35].

Within the cutaneous inflammatory pathologies, the entity of hidradenitis suppurativa deserves a separate chapter (Chap. 3), which is an entity that affects the apocrine glands of the body [36], generally chronic, debilitating with sequelae that can severely limit the quality of life of the patients who suffer it and be devastating for their self-esteem or be associated not infrequently with suicidal attempts. At present, with the approval of the use of biological drugs for treatment, it has been possible to modify the course of the disorder; therefore, it is of vital importance to make a timely diagnosis and targeted treatment using high-resolution ultrasound that has proven to be more accurate than clinical inspection for the staging of the disease, including finding hidden lesions such as subdermal nodules, fistulas, complex multi-fistula-sinus tracts, and the presence of retained hair fragments [37–44] (Fig. 1.12). By means of the Doppler exploration, it is possible to quantitatively monitor the inflammatory activity of the disease and to carry out a more objective follow-up of the efficacy of the treatments [1, 45].

wood and fish bones [46, 47]. In ultrasound, they are observed as a laminar, hyperechoic band that is usually associated with surrounding hypoechoic mass due to the development of granuloma in the periphery (Fig. 1.13). Elements such as glass or metal can be better identified by the presence of the reverberation artifact. Postsurgical granulomas develop due to non-absorbable surgical material with a typical appearance of a markedly hypoechoic nodule with a defined hyperechoic linear center (Fig. 1.14). Ultrasound can confirm the presence of a foreign body, the type of element, and its exact location that helps to extract it under ultrasound image guidance.

1.6 Identification of Foreign Bodies

Depending on their nature, foreign bodies are classified as inert corresponding to glass, metal, postsurgical, or organic material corresponding to

1.7 Traumatic Pathology and Sequelae

The usefulness of ultrasound in traumatic musculoskeletal lesions is well known and can clarify complications and sequelae of injury such as the presence of hematomas, seromas, and post-traumatic fibrosis and the development of fistulous tracts and hypertrophic scars.

The appearance of post-trauma collections is one of the most frequent reasons for ultrasound examination where hematomas or seromas develop. Bruises contain red blood cells, clots, and inflammatory cells in the acute phase and, in the late phases, granulation tissue and fibrin. Patients with hemophilia, Ehler-Danlos syndrome, and anticoagulants develop soft tissue hematomas very easily [48]. In ultrasound, their appearance varies according to the evolution phase and the presence of liquefaction changes usually presenting as well-defined anechoic collections that become hypo- and hyperechoic over time (Fig. 1.14). In the early stages, they may show hypervascularization in the periphery at Doppler exploration and hypovascularity in the late phases [49]. Seromas or lymphoceles are composed mainly of clear lymphatic fluid produced by tearing in the lymphatic network commonly seen after cosmetic surgical procedures such as tummy tucks (Fig. 1.15). A fistula is a pathological communication path between two anatomical spaces or a path that leads from the internal cavity of an organ to the surface of the skin. Usually they originate from an infectious process of the deep layers that tries to drain to the surface. Clinically they present as an erythematous or ulcerated spot or nodule with discharge of material that may be serous, purulent, or hematic. Ultrasound shows a hypoechoic tract, usually linear, of variable diameter with internal echoes and Doppler scanning vascularization in the periphery (Fig. 1.16).

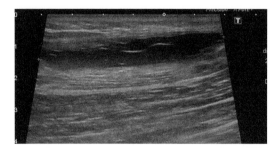

Fig. 1.15 Image with a lentiform configuration, with some echoes in its interior, corresponding to a hematoma of slugged evolution

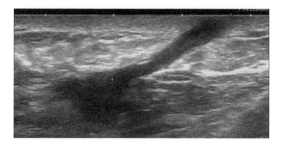

Fig. 1.16 Typical image of sinus fistula with oblique orientation that connects small collection in subcutaneous cellular tissue with the surface

1.8 Conclusion

High-resolution ultrasound is a useful tool that allows to make an adequate diagnosis of many dermatological lesions; it is possible to establish if the lesion is of skin or not, its precise extension, the solid or cystic content of the lesion, and its degree of vascularization; and it provides additional information to the clinician for its management.

References

1. Wortsman X, Wortsman J. Clinical usefulness of variable frequency ultrasound in localized lesions of the skin. J Am Acad Dermatol. 2010;62:247–56.
2. Wortsman X, Jemec GB. Dermatological Ultrasound with clinical and histologic correlation. 1st ed. New York: Springer; 2013.
3. Cammarota T, Pinto F, Magliaro A, et al. Current uses of diagnostic high frequency US in dermatology. Eur J Radiol. 1998;27:215–23.
4. Antoch G, Vongt FM, Freudengerg LS, et al. Whole body dual modality PET/CT and whole body MRI for staging in oncology. JAMA. 2003;290:3199–206.
5. Wortsman X. The traces of sound: taking the road to skin. Curr Rheumatol Rev. 2011;7:2–8.
6. Szymańska E, Nowichcki A, Mlosek K, et al. Skin imaging with high frequency ultrasound: preliminary results. Eur J Ultrasound. 2000;12:9–16.
7. Wortsman X. Common applications of dermatologic sonography. J Ultrasound Med. 2012;31:97–111.
8. Wortsman X, Wortsman J, Arellano J, Oroz J, Guigliano C, Benavides MI, Bordon C. Pilomatrixomas presenting as vascular tumors on color Doppler ultrasound. J Pediatr Surg. 2010;45:2094–8.
9. Kanitakis J. Anatomy, histology and immunohistochemistry of normal human skin. Eur J Dermatol. 2002;12:3900–9.

10. Proksch E, Brandner JM, Jensen JM. The skin: an indispensable barrier. Exp Dermatol. 2008;17:1063–72.
11. Ebling FJG, Eady RA, Leigh IM. Anatomy and organization of human skin. In: Rook AJ, Wilkinson DS, Ebling FJG, editors. Textbook of dermatology. Oxford: Blackwell Scientific Publications; 1992. p. 49.
12. Ghianidecka M, Ghianidecka R, Serup J, et al. Ultrasound structure and digital image analysis of subdermal low echogenic band in aged human skin: diurnal changes and inter individual variability. J Invest Dermatol. 1994;102:362–5.
13. Huang C-C, Ko S-F, Huang H-Y, Ng S-H, Lee T-Y, Lee Y-W, Chen M-C. Epidermal cysts in the superficial soft tissue: sonography features with an emphasis on the pseudotestis pattern. Ultrasound Med. 2011;30:11–7.
14. Solivetti FM, Elia F, Drusco A, et al. Epithelioma of Malherbe: new ultrasound patterns. J Exp Clin Cancer Res. 2010;29:42.
15. Choo HJ, Lee SJ, Lee YH, Lee JH, Oh M, Kim MH, Lee EJ, Song JW, Kim SJ, Kim DW. Pilomatricomas: the diagnostic value of ultrasound. Skeletal Radiol. 2010;39:243–50.
16. Roche NA, Monstrey SJ, Matton GE. Pilomatricoma in children common but often misdiagnosed. Acta Chir Belg. 2010;110:250–4.
17. Hwang JY, Lee SM. The common ultrasonography features of Pilomatricoma. J Ultrasound Med. 2005;24:1397–402.
18. Hsu YC, Shih YY, Gao HW, et al. Subcutaneous lipoma compression de common nerve as causing palsy: sonography diagnosis. J Clin Ultrasound. 2010;38:97–9.
19. Inampudi P, Jacobson JA, Fessell DP, et al. Soft tissue lipomas: accuracy of sonography in diagnosis with pathologic diagnosis. Radiology. 2004;233:763–7.
20. Yang DM, Kim HC, Lim JW, et al. Sonography findings of groin masses. J Ultrasound Med. 2007;26:605–14.
21. Fornage BD, Tassin GB. Sonography appearances of superficial soft tissue lipomas. J Clin Ultrasound. 1991;19:215–20.
22. Kuwano Y, Ishizaki K, Watanabe R, Nanko H. Efficacy of diagnostic ultrasonography of lipomas, epidermal cysts, and ganglions. Arch Dermatol. 2009;145:761–4.
23. Harlak A, Mentes O, Kilic S, et al. Sacrococcygeal pilonidal disease: analysis of previously proposed risk factors. Clinics (Sao Paulo). 2010;65:125–31.
24. Mentes O, Oysul A, Harlak A, Zeybek N, Kozak O, Tufan T. Ultrasonography accurately evaluates the dimension and shape of the pilonidal sinus. Clinics (Sao Paulo). 2009;64:189–92.
25. Gidwaney R, Bradley L, Yam B, et al. Endometriosis of abdominal and pelvic wall scars: multimodality imaging findings, pathologic correlation and radiologic mimics. Radiographics. 2012;32(7):2031–43.
26. Al-Khateeb TH, Al-Masri NM, Al-Zoubi F. Cutaneous cysts of the head and neck. J Oral Maxillofac Surg. 2009;67:52–7.
27. Kirwan LA. Dermoid cyst of the lateral third of eyebrow. Practitioner. 1985;229:771–3.
28. Choudur HN, Hunjan JS, Howey JM, et al. Unusual presentation of dermal cyst in the ischiorectal fossa. Magnetic resonance imaging and ultrasound appearances. Skeletal Radiol. 2009;38:291–4.
29. Nocini P, Barbaglio A, Dolci M, et al. Dermoid cysts of the nose: a case report and review of the literature. J Oral Maxillofac Surg. 1996;54:357–62.
30. Smirniotopoulus JG, Chiechi MV. Teratomas, dermoids, and epidermoids of the head and neck. Radiographics. 1995;15:1437–62.
31. Restrepo S, Lemos D, Gordillo H, et al. Imaging findings in musculoskeletal complications of AIDS. Radiographics. 2004;24:1029–49.
32. Fayad L, Carrino J, Fishman L, et al. Musculoskeletal infection: role of CT in the emergency department. Radiographics. 2007;27:1723–36.
33. Ebrigth JR, Pieper B. Skin and soft tissue infections in drug users. Infect Dis Clin North Am. 2002;16:697–712.
34. Latifi HR, Siegerl MJ. Color Doppler flow imaging in pediatric soft tissue masses. J Ultrasound Med. 1994;13:165–9.
35. Nonh JY, Cheong HJ, Hongh SJ, et al. Skin and soft tissue infections experience over a five year period and clinical usefulness of ultrasonography gun biopsy-based culture. Scand J Infect Dis. 2011;43:870–6.
36. Von der Werth JM, Williams HC. The natural history of hidradenitis suppurativa. J Eur Acad Dermatol Venereol. 2000;14:389–92.
37. Wortsman X. Imaging of hidradenitis suppurativa. Dermatol Clin. 2016;34(1):59–68.
38. Martorell A, Segura Palacios JM. Ultrasound examination of hidradenitis suppurativa. Actas Dermosifiliogr. 2015;106(Suppl 1):49–59.
39. Wortsman X, Rodriguez C, Lobos C, Eguiguren G. Ultrasound diagnosis and staging in pediatric hidradenitis suppurativa. Pediatr Dermatol. 2016;33(4): e260–4. https://doi.org/10.1111/pde.12895.. Epub 2016 Jun 13
40. Wortsman X, Jemec G. A 3D ultrasound study of sinus tract formation in hidradenitis suppurativa. Dermatol Online J. 2013;19:18564.
41. Wortsman X, Jemec GBE. Real-time compound imaging ultrasound of hidradenitis suppurativa. Dermatol Surg. 2007;33:1340–2.
42. Jemec GBE, Gniadecka M. Ultrasound examination of hair follicles in hidradenitis. Arch Dermatol. 1997;133:967–72.
43. Wortsman X, Wortsman J. Ultrasound detection of retained hair tracts in hidradenitis suppurativa. Dermatol Surg. 2015;41:867–9.
44. Wortsman X, Revuz J, Jemec GB. Lymph nodes in hidradenitis suppurativa. Dermatology. 2009;219:22–4.
45. Martorell A, Worstman X, Alfagame F, Roustan G, Arias-Santiago S, Catalano O, Scotto di Santolo M, Zarchi K, Bouer M, Gattini D, Gonzalez C, Bard R, Garcia-Martínez FJ, Mandava A. Ultrasound evaluation

as a complementary test in hidradenitis suppurativa: proposal of a standardized report. Dermatol Surg. 2017;43(8):1065–73.

46. Soudack M, Nachtigal Λ, Gaitini D. Clinically unsuspected foreign bodies: the importance of sonography. J Ultrasound Med. 2003;22:1381–5.

47. Wortsman X. Sonography of cutaneous and ungual lumps and Bumps. Ultrasound Clin. 2012;7:505–23.

48. Hermann G, Gilbert MS, Abdelwahab IF. Hemophilia: evaluation of musculoskeletal involvement with CT, sonography and MR imaging. AJR Am J Roengenol. 1992;158:119–23.

49. Sidhu PS, Rich PM. Sonography detection and characterization of musculoskeletal and subcutaneous tissue abnormalities in sickle cell disease. Br J Radiol. 1999;72:9–17.

Image-Guided Treatments in Skin Inflammatory Diseases

Fernando Alfageme

2.1 Introduction

Inflammatory skin conditions can be, in general terms, the result of an infectious or non-infectious disease. Within this last group, psoriasis, hidradenitis suppurativa, and rheumatologic diseases stand out as the most common pathologies.

Cutaneous ultrasound can provide information on the extension of the inflammation and also follow eventual complications that may arise from that inflammation, thus becoming a very useful tool to monitor the treatments prescribed to the patients.

2.2 Basic Principles of Ultrasound of Cutaneous Inflammatory Diseases

Pathophysiologically any skin inflammation disorder is accompanied by an increase in the blood flow of the affected area [1]. The superficial vascular plexus, found in the dermoepidermal junction, is the structure with the highest capacity of intravascular and extravascular exchange (Fig. 2.1).

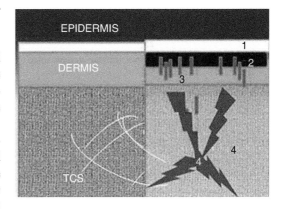

Fig. 2.1 Ultrasound findings of inflammatory diseases. (*1*) Epidermal thickening, (*2*) dermal hypoechogenicity, (*3*) increased vascularization, (*4*) subcutaneous tissue cobblestone pattern. TCS-fatty tissue

Given this, the first sign of inflammation that is visible in ultrasound is the increase in the vascular flow of the affected area, compared to the flow registered in surrounding areas [2].

This increased flow leads to the accumulation of intravascular serum and mediator inflammation cells and mediators. This phenomenon is characterized in ultrasound as hypoechogenicity of the superficial dermal band which corresponds anatomically to papillary dermis [1].

If the inflammatory infiltrate reaches the subcutaneous tissue, increased vascular flow in this tissue will be observed together with this being identifiable hypoechogenicity of the interlobular septa and the changes in echogenicity of fatty

F. Alfageme (✉)
Dermatologic Ultrasound Learning Centre
(EFSUMB), Hospital Universitario Puerta de Hierro
Majadahonda Madrid, Universidad Autónoma de
Madrid, Madrid, Spain

R. L. Bard (ed.), *Image Guided Dermatologic Treatments*,
https://doi.org/10.1007/978-3-030-29236-2_2

lobules [3] which increases echogenicity in *a cobblestone pattern*.

If the vascular inflammation becomes very intense, it can lead to necrosis which is characterized in ultrasound images as hypoechoic and unstructured areas in dermis or subcutaneous tissue associated with decreased beam penetration and resolution.

Reparation processes after inflammatory events of the skin are characterized by the replacement of inflamed tissue by a scar [2] (mainly composed of collagen) that is hypoechogenic in the first stages and then becomes hyperechogenic when the contraction and remodeling process is completed.

2.3 Ultrasound of Skin Infectious Diseases

Microbial infection (caused by viruses, bacteria, or fungi) of the skin is normally accompanied by an inflammation of the infected layer. Viruses often infect more superficial layers of the skin. The viral infections better characterized from the sonographic point of view are those caused by human papillomavirus (HPV).

HPV type 1 affects mainly plantar surfaces, and the infection is characterized by an inflammation of both superficial and deep tissues (Fig. 2.2). The second histologic feature of HPV infection is hyperkeratosis of superficial layers. The inflammatory process is accompanied by inflammation of deeper structures such as the joint bursae [4]. In this sense, ultrasonography becomes very useful for the diagnosis of plantar warts and to guide further treatment in recalcitrant cases. Since warts are vascular, they may be mistaken for malignant melanoma varieties; however, wart generally has a central vertical vascular supply, while melanoma is diffuse and lateral in vessel pattern.

Cryotherapy, ablative procedures, and vascular laser are efficient treatment modalities in which ultrasound indicates if inflammation is progressively decreasing from the deep to the superficial layers as a measure of success.

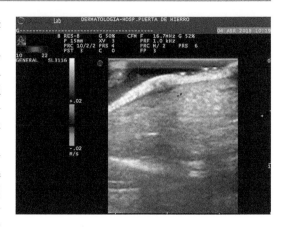

Fig. 2.2 Plantar wart. Epidermal thickening with hypoechogenicity of dermis and increased vascularization indicates inflammation and necessity of cryosurgery or laser therapy

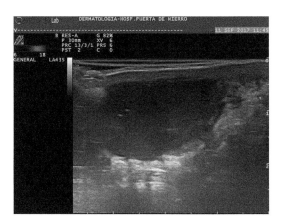

Fig. 2.3 Abscess. Well-defined hypoechoic area with internal debris indicates the need of surgical drainage

The reaction of the body to an inflammation caused by *bacterial infection* is frequently the isolation of the focus of the infection through the formation of pyogenic abscesses. These may not be clinically evident, which is problematic because they need drainage to be treated and may enlarge or rupture causing locoregional inflammation and necrosis [5, 6]. Ultrasound clearly defines the abscess limits (Fig. 2.3), which is essential to guide the incision and drainage process.

Regarding mycoses, ultrasound is useful in the differential diagnosis of onychomycoses (Fig. 2.4) from psoriatic onycopathy [7].

In the case of psoriasis, ventral thickening of nail plate is evident in contrast with onychomycoses in which dorsal plate involvement is also present. Nail plate thickness over 1 mm suggests that topical therapies will have lessened clinical effect due to penetration issues. Together with increased vascularization of the nail bed in psoriasis, this sonographic difference is relevant to prescribe antifungal drugs which are not exempt from the secondary effects of high potency corticosteroids which are the keystone treatment for nail psoriasis along with the immunologic therapies.

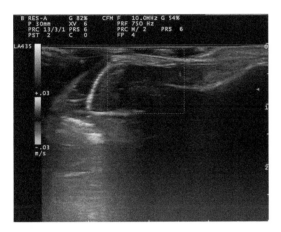

Fig. 2.4 Onychomycosis. Diffuse thickening of nail plate without increased vascularization of the nail bed. In this case oral antifungal is necessary due to full nail plate involvement

2.4   Non-infectious Inflammatory Skin Diseases: Psoriasis

Psoriasis is nowadays considered a systemic inflammatory disease that affects the skin, nails, and joints. It has recently been shown to diffusely involve the cardiovascular system as the vasculitis process continues unchecked.

Methods used to quantify the extent or severity of skin psoriasis (PASI-NAPSI) are subjective and highly susceptible to interobserver variation. These variations make early psoriasis detection and treatment follow-up difficult to evaluate [8].

Ultrasound of the psoriatic plaque follows the same general ultrasonographic principles of skin inflammation:

1. Dermoepidermal thickening
2. Appearance of hypoechoic band in the superficial dermis that correlates with inflammation
3. Increased flow in the dermis visible with Doppler

Regarding nails, general features of psoriatic onycopathy are (Fig. 2.5):

- Thickening of the nail bed (measured from the table to the phalanx)
- Loss of definition of the ventral nail plate
- Increased flow in the nail bed

Fig. 2.5 Psoriatic nail clinical and sonographic images. In contrast with onychomycoses, ventral plate involvement and increased nail bed vascularization are keys to differentiate them from onychomycoses

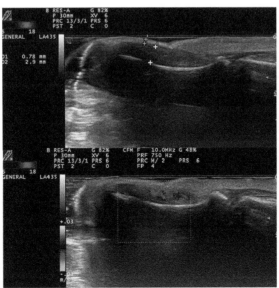
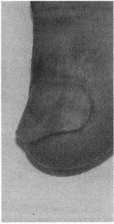

Ultrasonographic follow-up of topical and systemic treatments in psoriasis has proven to be sensitive for changes induced by the use of these treatments [9, 10].

2.5 Ultrasonography of Inflammatory Skin Diseases: Lupus, Dermatomyositis, and Morphea

This group of diseases has two phases: an active inflammatory phase and an atrophy-sclerosis phase [11].

Most rheumatologic skin diseases are best treated in the *active* inflammatory phase; therefore, the use of ultrasound to discriminate between these two phases is relevant above all in the case of deep sclerosing diseases in which clinical findings are usually inconclusive.

Active phase ultrasound findings in this group of diseases are [11]:

• Changes in epidermis
• Hypoechoic dermis
• Increased echogenicity of subcutaneous cellular tissue
• Increased flow at the dermis and at the subcutaneous cellular tissue (Fig. 2.6)

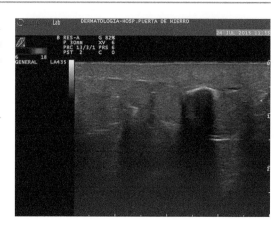

Fig. 2.7 Calcinosis in dermatomyositis, an indicator of ill prognosis

Dermatomyositis and systemic sclerosis can cause calcinosis, which is characterized by signs of calcification (hyperechoic, posterior acoustic shadowing) and vascular thrombosis. The appearance of both these signs indicates poor prognosis in these diseases (Fig. 2.7).

Inactive or atrophic phase ultrasonographic findings in rheumatological diseases are:

• Thinning of the dermis and of subcutaneous tissue
• Increase of the fibrous component in the dermis and hypodermis
• Decreased vascularization

New ultrasonographic techniques such as electrography [12] are being used to assess skin sclerosing diseases in the atrophic phase (Fig. 2.8).

2.6 Ultrasonography in Hidradenitis Suppurativa

Hidradenitis suppurativa (HS) is an immune-mediated disease targeting follicles in the apocrine areas of the body (axillae, groin, gluteal, inframammary) [13].

This chronic debilitating disease is usually underestimated due to the deep location of the lesions that are felt by the patient but often are occult to the naked eye.

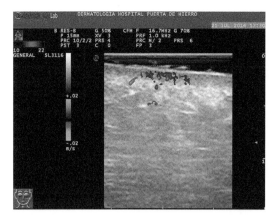

Fig. 2.6 Acute lupus, active phase; increased vascularization observed

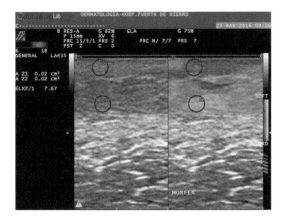

Fig. 2.8 Morphea. B mode and strain elastography. Increased strain is evident in dermal subdermal junction indicating severe sclerosis

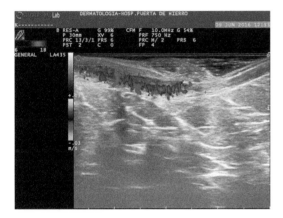

Fig. 2.9 Axillary fistulous tract in a patient with HS. Active inflammation evidenced by hypervascularization of the tract indicates need for systemic treatment (biological, antibiotic therapy)

The role of ultrasound in the management of this disease is key to fully avoid irreversible atrophic scars that may lead to functional impairment and social exclusion due to foul discharge of the structurally established lesions.

According to Wortsman et al., three types of active evolutive lesions can be observed in HS [14]

1. *Pseudocyst:* Limited hypoechoic area in dermis
2. *Fistulous tracts:* Linear dermal-subdermal areas that connect several follicles (Fig. 2.9)
3. *Fluid collections:* Subdermal hypoechoic areas or purulent content

Adequate treatment of HS depends mainly in sonographic staging according to these lesions. While as pseudocysts may be treated with lasers or topical antibiotics, fistulae or collections indicate the need of a systemic or combined surgical treatment.

References

1. Wortsman X, Jemec G. Common inflammatory diseases of the skin: From the skin to the screen. Adv Psoriasis Inflammatory Skin Dis. 2010;2:9–15.
2. Alfageme F. Ultrasound skin imaging. Actas Dermosifiliogr. 2014;105:891–9.
3. Iverson K, Haritos D, Thomas R, Kannikeswaran N. The effect of bedside ultrasound on diagnosis and management of soft tissue infections in a pediatric ED. Am J Emerg Med. 2012;30:1347–51.
4. Wortsman X, Jemec GBE, Sazunic I. Anatomical detection of inflammatory changes associated to plantar warts. Dermatology. 2010;220:213–7.
5. Ramirez-Schrempp D, Dorfman DH, Baker W, Liteplo AS. Ultrasound soft-tissue applications in the pediatric emergency department: to drain or not to drain? Pediatr Emerg Care. 2009;25:44–8.
6. Squire BT, Fox JC, Anderson C. ABSCESS: applied bedside sonography for convenient evaluation of superficial soft tissue infections. Acad Emerg Med. 2005;12:601–6.
7. Gutierrez M, Wortsman X, Filippucci E, de Angelis R, Filosa G, Grassi W. High-frequency sonography in the evaluation of psoriasis: nail and skin involvement. J Ultrasound Med. 2009;28:1569–74.
8. Gutierrez M, Filippucci E, Bertolazzi C, Grassi W. Sonographic monitoring of psoriatic plaque. J Rheumatol. 2009;36:850–1.
9. Gutierrez M, de Angelis R, Bernardini ML, Filippucci E, Goteri G, Brandozzi G, et al. Clinical, power Doppler sonography and histological assessment of the psoriatic plaque: short-term monitoring in patients treated with etanercept. Br J Dermatol. 2011;164:33–7.
10. Lacarrubba F, Nardone B, Musumeci ML, Micali G. Ultrasound evaluation of clobetasol propionate 0.05% foam application in psoriatic and healthy skin: a pilot study. Dermatol Ther. 2009;22(Suppl 1):S19–21.
11. Wortsman X, Wortsman J, Sazunic I, Carreño L. Activity assessment in morphea using color doppler ultrasound. J Am Acad Dermatol. 2011;65:942–8.
12. Alfageme Roldán F. Elastography in dermatology. Actas Dermosifiliogr. 2016;107:652–60.
13. Wortsman X, Jemec GBE. High frequency ultrasound for the assessment of hidradenitis suppurativa. Dermatol Surg. 2007;33:1–3.
14. Kelekis NL, Efstathopoulos E, Balanika A, Spyridopoulos TN, Pelekanou A, Kanni T, et al. Ultrasound aids in diagnosis and severity assessment of hidradenitis suppurativa. Br J Dermatol. 2010;1:1400–2.

Ultrasound of Hidradenitis Suppurativa

3

Raffaele Dante Caposiena Caro

3.1 Introduction

Hidradenitis suppurativa (HS), also known as acne inversa or Verneuil disease, is a chronic, inflammatory, recurrent, debilitating skin disease of the terminal hair follicle, usually presenting after puberty with painful, deep-seated, inflamed lesions in the apocrine gland-bearing areas of the body, most commonly the axillary, inguinal, and anogenital regions [1–4].

3.2 Epidemiology

3.2.1 Incidence

The exact incidence of HS remains unknown. Vazquez et al. found an annual age- and sex-adjusted incidence of 6.0 per 100,000 person-years, with a higher incidence rate among women (8.2 per 100,000) compared to men (3.8 per 100,000) [5]. The highest incidence of HS for both women and men was between 20 and 29 years of age (18.4 and 7.4 per 100,000, respectively). The incidence of HS progressively declines with increasing age, especially in women older than 49 years old maybe due in part to the onset of menopause [6, 7].

3.2.2 Prevalence

Similarly, the prevalence of HS is not widely elucidated. Recently, Ingram et al. found a prevalence of 0.77% in the UK, while in Europe, it is estimated at 1% in the general population and at 4% in young adult women [8–11]. The overall HS prevalence in the US population sample was 98 per 100,000, while the adjusted prevalence in women was 137 per 100,000, more than twice that of men (58 per 100,000), and higher among patients aged 30–39 years (172 per 100,00) [12]. In an Australian study, a prevalence rate of 0.67% was found [13].

3.3 Pathogenesis

The etiopathogenesis of HS is not fully understood. Current evidence highlights a complex multifactorial pathogenesis [14].

3.3.1 Genetics

Genetic factors have been demonstrated only in a limited number of patients [15, 16]. Loss-of-function mutations of nicastrin (NCSTN) gene,

R. D. Caposiena Caro (✉)
Department of Systems Medicine, University of Rome, Tor Vergata, Rome, Italy

© Springer Nature Switzerland AG 2020
R. L. Bard (ed.), *Image Guided Dermatologic Treatments*,
https://doi.org/10.1007/978-3-030-29236-2_3

encoding key components of the γ-secretase, have been demonstrated; γ-secretase is a family of proteins that activates the Notch signaling pathway, affecting the expression of genes involved in epidermal cell and hair follicle differentiation and proliferation [15–18]. Other genes implicated in HS are PSTPIP1, IL-12Rb1, CDKAL1, MEFV, NLRP3, NLRP12, NOD2, LPIN2, and LCN2 [16–18].

3.3.2 Inflammation

Initially the lymphocytic infiltration is predominated by T cells [19] and then neutrophils, histiocytes, and additional lymphocytes are recruited through chemotaxis [20]. In later stages the inflammation is driven by mast cells, CD3+ and CD4+ T cells, CD20+ and CD138+ B cells, as well as CD11c+, CD14+, and CD68+ cells [21, 22]. Levels of TNF-α, IL-1β, IL-6, CXCL-8/IL-8, IL-10, IL-12p70, IL-17/IL-17A, IL-32, and IL-36/IL-36a/IL-36b/IL-36g were all found to be significantly higher when compared to controls [16, 23–29]. In addition, serum concentration of C-reactive protein (CRP) is elevated compared to healthy volunteers and associated with neutrophil count and HS disease severity [16, 27, 30].

3.3.3 Microbiome

HS is not an infectious disease, although inflammation, suppuration, and malodorous discharge, normally associated with bacterial infections, are clinical features of this disease. There are many studies that evidence the involvement of microbes in the disease pathogenesis. Biofilms have been identified in 67% of chronic lesions samples and in 75% of perilesional samples [31]. Additionally, microbiome differs significantly from that in healthy controls and varies with disease severity. The 68.8% of patients with both aerobic and anaerobic bacteria had the most severe grade of HS (Hurley stage III) [32, 33].

3.3.4 Physiological and Environmental Factors

Several studies support, in HS, the involvement of physiological and environmental factors, such as smoking, obesity, mechanical friction, and endocrinology [34–49]. Most of HS patients are smokers or ex-smokers; nicotine has been shown to cause hyperplasia of infundibular keratinocytes, activation of immune cells, induction of pro-inflammatory cytokines, reduced release of AMP, and enhanced cellular adhesion of bacteria, promoting the formation of biofilms [20]. Also obesity increases the levels of pro-inflammatory cytokines worsening the course of HS [38–42]. In addition, obesity might influence HS pathogenesis due to wider skin folds, increased perspiration, local sweat retention, and enhanced friction promoting the "Koebner phenomenon" [43]. Finally, the female sex preponderance suggests that hormones may be pathogenically important. However, to date the exact role of sex hormones remains unknown [38, 44–48].

In conclusion, the first event is the follicular occlusion, maybe due to endogenous factors (as genetic) and/or exogenous factors (such as smoke, obesity mechanical stress), with subsequent dilatation of the hair follicle. Moreover, follicular occlusion may induce microbial dysbiosis and altered keratinocytes homeostasis. The second event is the dilated follicle rupture with releasing of keratin fibers, hair fragments, and bacteria to the surrounding tissue which induces a simultaneous activation of multiple inflammatory pathways, followed by foreign body type-like inflammation, with a diverse cell infiltrate, leading to an erythematous nodule or fluctuating abscess formation. Finally, the presence of epithelial strands in the dermis, imbalance in matrix metalloproteinases and tissue inhibitors of metalloproteinase, and increased activity of fibrotic factors may lead to the development of fistulae (tunnels) and scarring, a hallmark of chronic HS. Draining tunnels provide an excellent habitat for biofilm producing bacteria, which are able to continuously trigger inflammation with associated purulent drainage [16].

3.4 Clinical Features with Ultrasound Correlation

Clinically, it shows a wide spectrum of cutaneous lesions, often in diverse stages of evolutions [49]. However, physical examination may not detect inflammatory lesions such as nodules and abscesses, or fistulous tracts, which are critical data to assess the HS severity [50]. Additionally, the difference between a draining abscess and a draining tunnel or the real extent of inflammatory edema is clinically difficult to be recognized. Wortsman et al. [51] and Martorell et al. [52] showed in two different studies that clinical examination alone usually underestimates the severity of HS. Ultrasound is a useful tool to diagnose and stage correctly HS, detecting inflammatory lesions and/or fistulous tracts, all findings that may require a change in the treatment [50]. Clinical and sonographic definitions of HS lesion are shown in Table 3.1 [51, 53].

The HS begins with follicular occlusion, with subsequent dilatation as visualized by ultrasound (Fig. 3.1a). Then the rupture of the dilated follicle leads to the formation of solitary or multiple nodules (pseudocysts), which average duration is 1–2 weeks, but sometimes they may persist even for months (Fig. 3.1b). Nodules may be painful and deep situated in the hypodermis making them sometimes barely observable. Patients may report prodromal symptoms, such as burning, stinging pain, itching, warmth, and/or hyperhidrosis 12–48 h before nodule arises. Then they may resolve spontaneously or persist "silently" with sporadic episodes of inflammation or, lastly, become abscesses with possible rupture and ooze of pus (Fig. 3.1c). Recurrence of lesions and continued inflammation may lead to draining tunnel formation with intermittent/continuous release of foul odorous serous, purulent, or bloodstained discharge (Fig. 3.1d). Without adequate medical and/or surgical excision, sinus tracts may persist for months or also years. Finally, chronic inflammation may result in the formation of uniporous or multiporous comedones and scars (atrophic or hypertrophic) [53, 54].

HS has a predilection for hair-bearing skin sites and, especially, for body regions with apocrine sweat glands; most characteristic affected areas are axillae, groins, perianal, perineal, mammary (Fig. 3.2), inframammary, buttocks, and pubis and less commonly chest, nape, and retroauricular areas. This distribution pattern corresponds for the most part with the "milk line" distribution of apocrine-related mammary tissue in mammals. Furthermore, different grades of severity, areas of involvement, complications, extra-cutaneous features such as arthritis, and constitutional symptoms (fever, sickness) may occur [53–56].

Table 3.1 Lesion type and definition

Type	Clinical definition	Ultrasound definition
Nodule (pseudocyst)	Raised lesion, round, diameter >10 mm, three-dimensional	Round- or oval-shaped hypoechoic or anechoic nodular dermal and/or hypodermal structure
Abscess (fluid collection)	Swelling lesion, three-dimensional containing fluid (pus)	Hypoechoic or anechoic fluid dermal and/or hypodermal deposits connected to the base of widened hair follicles
Fistulous tract (tunnel)	Opening of variable length and depth, ending at the skin surface, and sometimes oozing a fluid	Hypoechoic or anechoic band-like dermal or hypodermal structure dermal connected to the base of widened hair follicles
Complex fistula (multitunnel)	The presence of numerous tunnels in a localized skin area; almost always, these tunnels may be interconnected	Two or more connected fistulous tracts in the same region

Wortsman et al. [51] and Lipsker et al. [53] modified

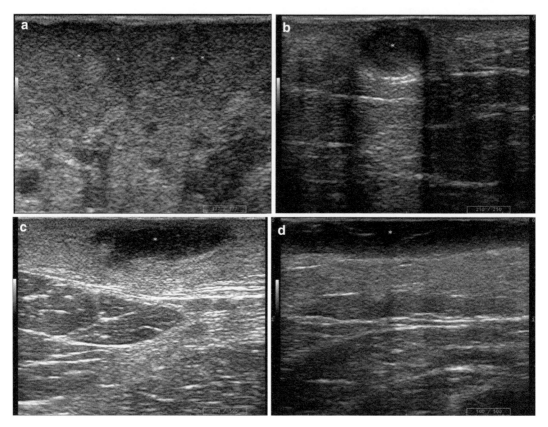

Fig. 3.1 (a) Widening of the hair follicles (∗) and thickening of the dermis. (b) Hypoechoic round-or oval-shaped nodule (pseudocyst) structure (∗) in the dermis and upper hypodermis with posterior acoustic reinforcement. (c) Hypoechoic collection (∗) with echoes (debris) and irregular borders in the dermis and upper hypodermis. (d) Ultrasound image (longitudinal view) hypoechoic fistulous tract (∗) running in the dermis

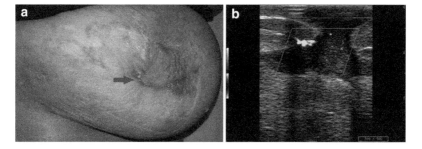

Fig. 3.2 (a) Hurley III patient with involvement of the left breast, draining tunnel (red arrow) with scar formation and retraction of the nipple. (b) Ultrasound correlation of figure (a) (red arrow) hypoechoic draining tunnel (∗) with echoes (debris) in the dermis and hypodermis connected with the surface of the skin, power Doppler positive with high signal and mixed distribution

3.4.1 Diagnosis

Clinical diagnosis is based on the following three criteria, which must all be met, for establishing diagnosis: (1) the presence of typical lesions, including deep-seated painful nodules, and/or abscesses, and/or draining sinuses, and/or bridged scars; (2) typical topography, with predominant involvement of the axillae and groin; and (3) chronic course with multiple recurrences. Still, there is often clinical diagnostic delay, especially in mild cases [57]. On the other hand, sonographic criteria include (1) widening of hair follicles, (2) thickening or abnormal echogenicity of the dermis, (3) dermal pseudocystic nodules (round- or oval-shaped hypoechoic or anechoic nodular structures), (4) fluid collections (anechoic or hypoechoic fluid deposits, in the dermis or hypodermis connected to the base of widened hair follicles), and (5) fistulous tracts (anechoic or hypoechoic band-like structures across skin layers in the dermis or hypodermis connected to the base of widened hair follicles). The presence of three or more sonographic criteria may establish the diagnosis [51].

3.5   Staging

Currently, there are several clinical staging systems used in the evaluation of HS severity (Table 3.2) [58–64]. However, the most commonly used scoring systems are (1) Hurley score, (2) HS-Physician's Global Assessment (HS-PGA), (3) Hidradenitis Suppurativa Severity Score System (IHS4), and (4) Hidradenitis Suppurativa Clinical Response (HiSCR).

The Hurley score was proposed in 1989 by Hurley and classifies patients into three stages [58]:

- Stage I: Solitary/multiple, isolated abscess formation without scarring or sinus tracts (Fig. 3.3)

Table 3.2 Clinical staging and severity scales

Score
• Hurley staging system
• Modified Sartorius Score (MSS)
• HS-Physician's Global Assessment (HS-PGA)
• Acne Inversa Severity Index (AISI)
• Hidradenitis Suppurativa Severity Index (HSSI)
• Hidradenitis Suppurativa Severity Score System (IHS4)
• Hidradenitis Suppurativa Clinical Response (HiSCR)

- Stage II: Recurrent abscesses, single/multiple widely separated lesions, with sinus tract formation and cicatrization (Fig. 3.4)
- Stage III: Diffuse/broad involvement or multiple interconnected sinus tracts/abscesses across the entire area (Fig. 3.5)

The HS-PGA is frequently used to measure clinical improvement in pharmacological trials, and it is easy to use. It classifies HS severity counting the number of lesions in all skin areas (Table 3.3) [62].

The IHS4 is a validated dynamic score system to assess the severity of HS. The resulting IHS4 score is arrived at by the number of nodules (multiplied by 1) plus the number of abscesses (multiplied by 2) plus the number of draining tunnels (multiplied by 4). A total score of ≤3 signifies mild, 4–10 signifies moderate, and ≥11 signifies severe disease [63].

Instead, HiSCR is a clinical endpoint to evaluate therapeutic outcomes in patients with hidradenitis suppurativa. To reach it patients, with baseline total abscess and inflammatory nodule (AN count) count ≥3 and draining fistula ≤20, must achieve at least a 50% reduction in total AN count, with no increase in abscess count and no increase in draining fistula count relative to baseline [64].

Ultrasound may be useful to characterize the subclinical abnormalities providing sonographic diagnostic criteria, improving the staging, and monitoring of the disease. Thus a sonographic score system for HS (SOS-HS) has been proposed; it classifies patients into three stages [51]:

- Stage I: Single fluid collection and dermal changes (hypoechoic or anechoic pseudocystic nodules, widening of the hair follicles, alterations in the dermal thickness, or echogenicity) affecting a single body segment (e.g., axilla, groin, breast, buttock) (unilateral or bilateral) without fistulous tracts
- Stage II: Two to four fluid collections or a single fistulous tract with dermal changes affecting up to two body segments (unilateral or bilateral)

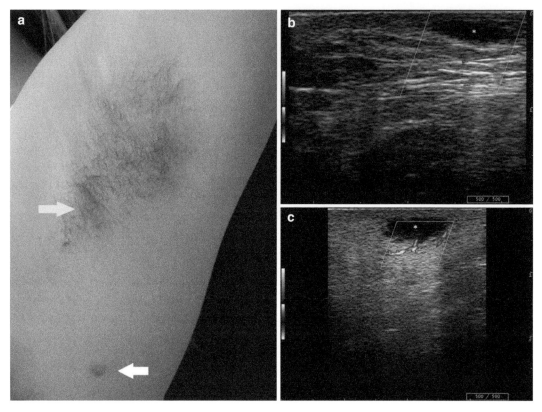

Fig. 3.3 (**a**) Nodular-abscess HS (Hurley I) of left axillar region. (**b**, **c**) Ultrasound correlation of figure (**a**) (white arrow) hypoechoic oval-shaped nodule (pseudocyst) structure (∗) in the dermis, power Doppler negative. (**c**) (Yellow arrow) hypoechoic collection (∗) with echoes (debris) and irregular borders in the dermis and upper hypodermis, power Doppler positive with high signal and peripheral distribution

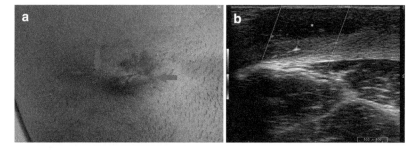

Fig. 3.4 (**a**) Hurley II patient with involvement of the right groin, draining tunnel with hypertrophic scar (blue arrow). (**b**) Ultrasound correlation of figure (**a**) (red arrow) hypoechoic draining tunnel (∗) with echoes (debris) in the dermis and hypodermis, power Doppler positive with high signal and mixed distribution

Fig. 3.5 (**a**) Hurley III patient with involvement of the left axilla. (**b–g**) Ultrasound correlation of figure (**a**). (**b**) (White arrow) hypoechoic oval-shaped nodule structure (∗) in the dermis; clinically also observable is a neighboring scar. (**c**) (Yellow arrow) hypoechoic collection (∗) with echoes (debris) and irregular borders in the dermis and upper hypodermis connected to the skin surface, power Doppler positive with moderate signal and peripheral distribution. (**d**) (Red circle) hypoechoic draining tunnel (∗) with echoes (debris) and irregular borders in the dermis and upper hypodermis (longitudinal view); notice the presence of a fragment of hair tracts and the three connections to the skin surface. (**e**) Power Doppler of the figure (**d**) moderate signal with mixed distribution. (**f**) (Red arrow) hypoechoic fistulous tract (∗) running in the dermis (longitudinal view). (**g**) (Blue arrow) hypoechoic fistulous tract (∗) running in the dermis (longitudinal view); clinically also observable is a neighboring scar

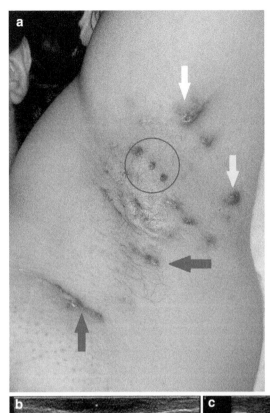

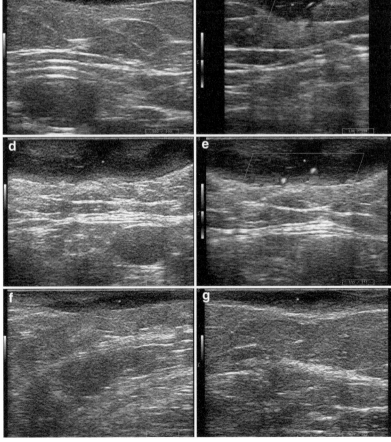

Table 3.3 HS-PGA scale

Stage	Description
Clear	No inflammatory or non-inflammatory nodules
Minimal	Only the presence of non-inflammatory nodules
Mild	Fewer than five inflammatory nodules or one abscess or draining fistula and no inflammatory nodules
Moderate	Fewer than 5 inflammatory nodules or 1 abscess or draining fistula and 1 or more inflammatory nodules or 2–5 abscesses or draining fistulas and fewer than 10 inflammatory nodules
Severe	Two to 5 abscesses or draining fistulas and 10 or more inflammatory nodules
Very severe	More than five abscesses or draining fistulas

Kimball et al. modified [62]

- Stage III: Five or more fluid collections or two or more fistulous tracts with dermal changes or involvement of three or more body segments (unilateral or bilateral)

Moreover, fistulous tracts can be classified according to the degree of fibrosis and edema [65]:

- Grading of fibrosis: 0 absent; 1 if present is a thin peripheral hypoechoic band (intermittent or continuous) with a fibrillar pattern; 2 if present is a thick and continuous peripheral hypoechoic band with a fibrillar pattern that invades the lumen of the tract and produces a hypoechoic "halo" sign in transverse view (intermittent or continuous)
- Grading of edema: 0 absent; 1 if present is a diffuse increase of the echogenicity of the hypodermis; 2 if present is a prominent hyperechoic hypodermal fatty lobules, with anechoic fluid between the fatty lobules

According to the grade of fibrosis and edema, fistulous tracts may be classified into three types [65]:

1. Low fibrotic scarring (grades 0–1) with high or low edema (grades 0–2) fistulous tract
2. High fibrotic scarring (grade 2) with low edema (grades 0–1) fistulous tract

3. High fibrotic scarring (grade 2) with high edema (grade 2)

Finally, color Doppler and power Doppler ultrasound may detect the presence of vascularity describing the blood flow patterns in real time. Nevertheless, power Doppler shows greater sensitivity compared to conventional color Doppler and is particularly helpful to investigate small vessels and those with low-velocity flow. Hypervascularity is a sign of active inflammation and so of active disease; consequently, its evaluation is a useful tool to monitor the degree of the inflammatory reaction and can add relevant information to assess disease severity and the response to therapies [66]. Power Doppler signal may be classified into (1) high if multiple flow signals are visible, (2) moderate if some flow signals are visible, (3) minimal if only few color spots are detectable, and (4) absent if no flow signal is identifiable [66]. Vascular distribution may be classified into three types [66]:

- Peripheral: the flow signals are predominantly at the periphery of the lesion.
- Internal: the flow signals are predominantly inside the lesion.
- Mixed: the flow signals are both at periphery and inside the lesion.

The presence vascularization inside the lesion is commonly due to the development of fibrotic and inflammatory tissue within the lesions [66].

3.6 Treatment

HS management consists in combined approaches and measures either preventive or medical or surgical [67]. A summary of all medical and surgical treatments is shown in Table 3.4.

3.6.1 Preventive Measures

There are lifestyle interventions that all patients will benefit, regardless of the clinical stage. The most important modifications include:

Table 3.4 Treatment guidelines

Severity	Medical treatments first line			Other therapies (second-third line)	Surgical and laser therapies
	Topical	Oral	Biologics		
PGA mild	Clindamycin (1%) BID for 12 weeks (GRADE B) Resorcinol (15%) QD—BID for flares as needed (GRADE C)	Tetracycline (500 mg) BID for 12 weeks (GRADE B) Doxycycline and minocycline (50–100 mg) BID (GRADE D)		Zinc salt 60–90 mg QD (GRADE C) Intralesional triamcinolone (3–5 mg) one time and then repeated monthly if necessary (GRADE D)	Excision or curettage of individual lesions (GRADE C) CO_2 and Nd:YAG laser therapy (GRADE A/C) Drainage of fluctuating abscesses (GRADE D)
PGA moderate		Tetracycline (500 mg) BID for 12 weeks (GRADE B) Doxycycline/ minocycline (50–100 mg) BID (GRADE D) Clindamycin (300 mg) + rifampicin (300 mg) combination BID for 10 weeks (GRADE B/C)	Adalimumab 160 mg week 0, 80 mg week 2, and then 40 mg weekly (GRADE A)	Rifampicin (10 mg/kg) QD + moxifloxacin (400 mg) QD + metronidazole (500 mg TID) for 12 weeks, with metronidazole discontinuation at week 6 (GRADE C) Dapsone (25–200 mg) QD (GRADE C/D) Acitretin (0.5 mg/kg) QD (GRADE C) Ertapenem 1 g iv QD for 6 weeks (GRADE C) Infliximab (5 mg/kg iv) on weeks 0, 2, and 6 and then every 8 weeks thereafter (GRADE B)	Excision or curettage of individual lesions (GRADE C) CO_2 and Nd:YAG laser therapy (GRADE A/C) Drainage of fluctuating abscesses (GRADE D) Deroofing of sinus tracts (GRADE C/D) STEEP surgery (GRADE C)
PGA severe— very severe		Clindamycin (300 mg) + rifampicin (300 mg) combination BID for 10 weeks (GRADE B/C)	Adalimumab 160 mg week 0, 80 mg week 2, and then 40 mg weekly (GRADE A)	Prednisone (40–60 mg) daily for 3–4 days and then taper (GRADE C/D) Cyclosporine (3–5 mg/kg) daily (GRADE C/D) Infliximab (5 mg/kg intravenous) on weeks 0, 2, and 6 and then every 8 weeks thereafter (GRADE B)	Total excision of the lesions and surrounding hair-bearing skin (GRADE B/C) Second intention healing (GRADE B) Primary closure (GRADE C) Reconstruction with Flap Plasty (GRADE A/B) Reconstruction with skin grafting and NPWT (GRADE C)

QD one time a day, *BID* two times a day, *TID* three times a day, *NPWT* Negative-pressure wound therapy, *CO_2* CO_2 ablative laser, *Nd:YAG* neodymium-doped yttrium aluminum garnet laser, *GRADE* grade of recommendation. A, high; B, moderate; C, low; D, very low. Saunte DML et al. modified [67], Gulliver W et al. [74] and Zouboulis CC et al. [75]

- Patients should be encouraged to avoid wearing tight-fitting clothing, in order to reduce heat and friction and thus inflammation and trauma.
- Smoker patients should be encouraged to stop; several case reports documenting HS improvement after smoking cessation have been published [34–38, 44, 68–70].
- Diet modification and weight loss should be recommended. Several studies show that excessive weight and dairy consumption of a high glycemic diet appear to exacerbate HS and reduce treatment response [38–42, 71–73].
- Psychological support as needed [67].

3.6.2   Medical Management

Medical treatment includes topical, oral, and biologic therapies [67].

3.6.3   Topical Therapies

Clindamycin lotion 1% is the only antibiotic that has been studied as a topical agent and is a first-line medication for HS patients with Hurley stage I or mild stage. It has antibacterial as well as anti-inflammatory activity [67, 74, 75]. Another topical treatment is 15% resorcinol; it has keratolytic and anti-inflammatory properties and may be used in patients with Hurley stages I and II [67, 74, 75].

3.6.4   Oral Antibiotics

Although HS is a chronic inflammatory skin disease, the first-line treatment option includes the use of oral antibiotics with anti-inflammatory properties, such as tetracyclines, dapsone, and the combination of clindamycin and rifampicin [67, 74, 75]. However, recently two studies showed the efficacy of clindamycin as monotherapy (Fig. 3.6) [73, 76]. Another possible antibiotic combination is rifampicin and moxifloxacin

and metronidazole that may be used in refractory patients [74, 75, 77]. Finally, intravenous ertapenem is an effective treatment to manage flares, as also reported by several studies [74, 75, 78–81]. Combination antibiotics carry an increased risk for potential drug-related adverse events, including diarrhea and *Clostridium difficile* infection [82]. Patients should also be made aware that rifampin causes orange discoloration to urine and other body secretions and has many known drug interactions [82].

3.6.5   Corticosteroids

Oral corticosteroids are useful to manage HS flare and may be an effective adjunct in recalcitrant HS. However, long-term corticosteroid treatment should be used with appropriate caution for the risk of adverse events [74, 75, 83]. Triamcinolone acetonide intralesion injections may be used to accelerate resolution of acute inflammatory lesions [74, 75, 83].

3.6.6   Biologics and Small Molecules

In case of failure to first-line treatment, biologic may be used. Among them the anti-TNFα adalimumab is the first-line biologic treatment for patients with moderate-to-severe disease and is the only biologic agent approved by the US Food and Drug Administration (FDA) and the European Medicines Agency (EMA) for the treatment of HS (Figs. 3.7 and 3.8) [84–87], whereas infliximab, ustekinumab, and anakinra are second- and third-line therapies. Recently, apremilast, an oral small molecule inhibitor of phosphodiesterase 4 (PDE4), showed a meaningful efficacy in HS patients [88]. Currently, several clinical trial phases II and III are ongoing using biologics including secukinumab (anti-IL17A), bimekizumab (dual anti-IL-17A and IL-17F), IFX-1 (anti-C5a), bermekimab (anti IL-1α), guselkumab (anti IL-23), and INCB054707 (JAK1 inhibitor) [89].

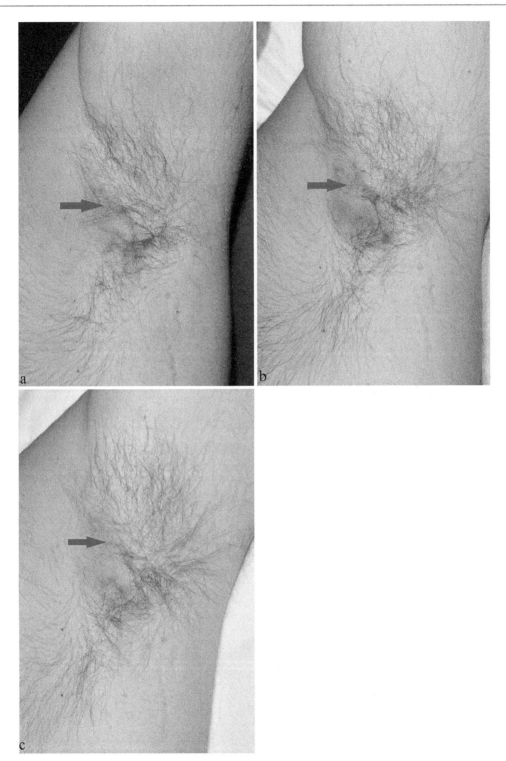

Fig. 3.6 (**a**) Hurley II patient with involvement of the left axilla, draining tunnel with (red arrow) baseline (T0). (**b**) After 2 months of treatment with clindamycin 300 BID mg (T8). (**c**) After 2 months of treatment with clindamycin 1% topical BID (T16). (**d–f**) Ultrasound correlations of picture (**a–c**). (**d**) Baseline (T0) (red arrow) hypoechoic fistulous tract (∗) running in the dermis (longitudinal view), power Doppler positive with minimal signal and peripheral distribution. (**e**) T8 (red arrow) hypoechoic fistulous tract (∗) running in the dermis (longitudinal view), power Doppler negative. (**f**) T16 slight thickening of the dermis

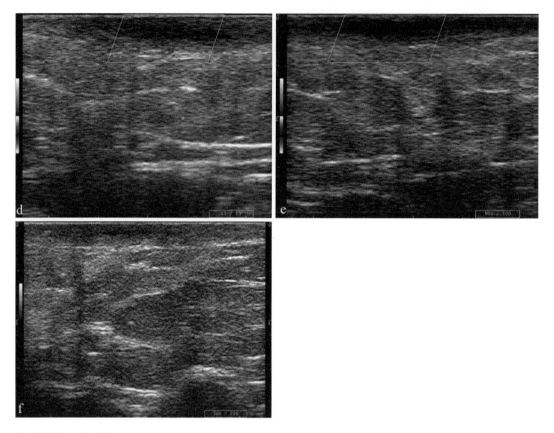

Fig. 3.6 (continued)

3.6.7 Retinoids

Acitretin and isotretinoin have been utilized in the treatment of HS [74, 75, 90, 91]. Especially systemic acitretin may be considered as a third-line therapy for patients with mild/moderate HS [91]. Isotretinoin has shown high value as a treatment of acne but less effective in HS [90, 92]. Retinoids are teratogenic and cannot be used in women who are pregnant or planning to become pregnant; in particular acitretin must be discontinued for at least 3 years prior to conception. Other side effects of this class of medication include xerosis, hyperlipidemia, and depression [93].

3.6.8 Other Therapies

Zinc salts with anti-inflammatory and anti-androgenic properties may be considered as a treatment option in Hurley I/II patients [74, 75].

Anti-androgenic therapies such as cyproterone acetate, oral contraceptive agents containing estrogen or norgestrel, and finasteride are other possible therapeutic options [94, 95]. Furthermore, anecdotal reports showed that spironolactone with its anti-androgenic activity may be an effective long-term agent [96].

3.6.9 Surgery and Light Laser Therapy

Surgery should be used in conjunction with lifestyle modifications and medical management. Several approaches can be used for solitary lesions such as limited excision, deroofing, and Skin-Tissue-sparing Excision with Electrosurgical Peeling (STEEP). They could be performed for recurrent HS lesions at fixed locations or fistula/sinus tract formation in limited areas. Instead, in Hurley III wide excision of the entire affected

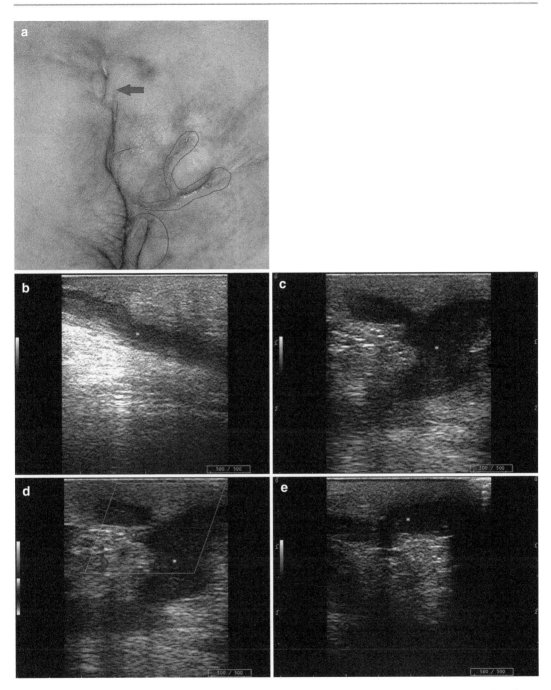

Fig. 3.7 (**a**) Hurley III patient with involvement of gluteus area at baseline. (**b–e**) Ultrasound correlations of picture (**a**). (**b**) (Red arrow) hypoechoic fistulous tract (∗) running in the dermis and hypodermis (longitudinal view). (**c**) (Continuous red line) hypoechoic draining multitunnel (∗) running in the dermis and deep penetrating in the hypodermis. (**d**) Power Doppler positive of the figure (**c**) with minimal signal and external distribution. (**e**) (Red circle) hypoechoic fistulous tract (∗) running in the dermis and hypodermis (longitudinal view). Caposiena Caro et al. modified [87]

Fig. 3.8 (**a**) Hurley III patient after 20 months of treatment with adalimumab. (**b**) (Red circle) hypoechoic fistulous tract (∗) running in the dermis and hypodermis (longitudinal view). Caposiena Caro et al. modified [87]

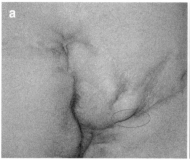
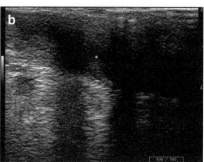

area may be performed to prevent recurrence. Furthermore, secondary intention healing revealed a lower risk of recurrences than primary closure or skin graft. In acute situations surgical incision and drainage of tense and painful lesions may be performed. However, incision and drainage should not be considered a cure because lesions treated with this technique usually recur. Effective alternative methods are CO_2 ablative laser and Nd:YAG laser; both showed a good efficacy and minimal patient discomfort in several studies [74, 75, 83].

References

1. Zouboulis CC, Del Marmol V, Mrowietz U, Prens EP, Tzellos T, Jemec GB. Hidradenitis suppurativa/acne inversa: criteria for diagnosis, severity assessment, classification and disease evaluation. Dermatology. 2015;231:184–90.
2. Plewig G, Steger M. Acne inversa (alias acne triad, acne tetrad or hidradenitis suppurativa). In: Marks R, Plewig G, editors. Acne and related disorders. London: Martin Dunitz; 1989. p. 345–57.
3. Von Laffert M, Helmbold P, Wohlrab J, et al. Hidradenitis suppurativa (acne inversa): early inflammatory events at terminal follicles and interfollicular epidermis. Exp Dermatol. 2010;19:533–7.
4. Fimmel S, Zouboulis CC. Comorbidities of hidradenitis suppurativa (acne inversa). Dermatol Endocrinol. 2010;2:9–16.
5. Vazquez BG, Alikhan A, Weaver AL, Wetter DA, Davis MD. Incidence of hidradenitis suppurativa and associated factors: a population-based study of Olmsted County, Minnesota. J Invest Dermatol. 2013;133:97–103.
6. Thornton JP, Abcarian H. Surgical treatment of perianal and perineal hidradenitis suppurativa. Dis Colon Rectum. 1978;21:573–7.
7. Fitzsimmons JS, Guilbert PR. A family study of hidradenitis suppurativa. J Med Genet. 1985;22:367–73.
8. Ingram JR, Jenkins-Jones S, Knipe DW, Morgan CLI, Cannings-John R, Piguet V. Population-based Clinical Practice Research Datalink study using algorithm modelling to identify the true burden of hidradenitis suppurativa. Br J Dermatol. 2018;178(4):917–24. https://doi.org/10.1111/bjd.16101.. Epub 2018 Feb 22.
9. Revuz JE, Canoui-Poitrine F, Wolkenstein P, et al. Prevalence and factors associated with hidradenitis suppurativa: results from two case-control studies. J Am Acad Dermatol. 2008;59:596–601.
10. Jemec GB, Heidenheim M, Nielsen NH. The prevalence of hidradenitis suppurativa and its potential precursor lesions. J Am Acad Dermatol. 1996;35:191–4.
11. Jemec GB. The symptomatology of hidradenitis suppurativa in women. Br J Dermatol. 1988;119:345–50.
12. Garg A, Lavian J, Lin G, Strunk A, Alloo A. Incidence of hidradenitis suppurativa in the United States: a sex- and age-adjusted population analysis. J Am Acad Dermatol. 2017;77(1):118–22.
13. Calao M, Wilson JL, Spelman L, Billot L, Rubel D, Watts AD, Jemec GBE. Hidradenitis Suppurativa (HS) prevalence, demographics and management pathways in Australia: a population-based cross-sectional study. PLoS One. 2018;13(7):e0200683. https://doi.org/10.1371/journal.pone.0200683.. eCollection 2018.
14. Banerjee A, Mcnish S, Shanmugam VK. Interferon-gamma (IFN-gamma) is elevated in wound exudate from hidradenitis suppurativa. Immunol Invest. 2017;46:149–58. https://doi.org/10.1080/08820139.2016.1230867.
15. Ingram JR. The genetics of hidradenitis suppurativa. Dermatol Clin. 2016;34(1):23–8. https://doi.org/10.1016/j.det.2015.07.002.
16. Vossen ARJV, van der Zee HH, Prens EP. Hidradenitis suppurativa: a systematic review integrating inflammatory pathways into a cohesive pathogenic model. Front Immunol. 2018;9:2965.
17. Starnes TW, Bennin DA, Bing X, Eickhoff JC, Grahf DC, Bellak JM, et al. The F-BAR protein PSTPIP1 controls extracellular matrix degradation and filopodia formation in macrophages. Blood. 2014;123:2703–14.

18. Zeeli T, Padalon-Brauch G, Ellenbogen E, Gat A, Sarig O, Sprecher E. Pyoderma gangrenosum, acne and ulcerative colitis in a patient with a novel mutation in the PSTPIP1 gene. Clin Exp Dermatol. 2015;40:367–72.

19. Boer J, Weltevreden EF. Hidradenitis suppurativa or acne inversa. A clinicopathological study of early lesions. Br J Dermatol. 1996;135(5):721–5.

20. Prens E, Deckers I. Pathophysiology of hidradenitis suppurativa: An update. J Am Acad Dermatol. 2015;73(5 Suppl 1):S8–11.

21. van der Zee HH, Laman JD, de Ruiter L, Dik WA, Prens EP. Adalimumab [antitumour necrosis factor alpha] treatment of hidradenitis suppurativa ameliorates skin inflammation: an in situ and ex vivo study. Br J Dermatol. 2012;166(2):298–305.

22. van der Zee HH, de Ruiter L, Boer J, et al. Alterations in leucocyte subsets and histomorphology in normal-appearing perilesional skin and early and chronic hidradenitis suppurativa lesions. Br J Dermatol. 2012;166(1):98–106.

23. Marzano AV, Damiani G, Ceccherini I, Berti E, Gattorno M, Cugno M. Autoinflammation in pyoderma gangrenosum and its syndromic form (pyoderma gangrenosum, acne and suppurative hidradenitis). Br J Dermatol. 2017;176:1588–98. https://doi.org/10.1111/bjd.15226.

24. Di Caprio R, Balato A, Caiazzo G, Lembo S, Raimondo A, Fabbrocini G, et al. IL-36 cytokines are increased in acne and hidradenitis suppurativa. Arch Dermatol Res. 2017;309:673–8. https://doi.org/10.1007/s00403-017-1769-5.

25. Thomi R, Kakeda M, Yawalkar N, Schlapbach C, Hunger RE. Increased expression of the interleukin-36 cytokines in lesions of hidradenitis suppurativa. J Eur Acad Dermatol Venereol. 2017;31:2091–6. https://doi.org/10.1111/jdv.14389.

26. Thomi R, Yerly D, Yawalkar N, Simon D, Schlapbach C, Hunger RE. Interleukin-32 is highly expressed in lesions of hidradenitis suppurativa. Br J Dermatol. 2017;177:1358–66. https://doi.org/10.1111/bjd.15458.

27. Jimenez-Gallo D, De La Varga-Martinez R, Ossorio-Garcia L, Albarran-Planelles C, Rodriguez C, Linares-Barrios M. The clinical significance of increased serum proinflammatory cytokines, C-reactive protein, and erythrocyte sedimentation rate in patients with hidradenitis suppurativa. Mediators Inflamm.2017;2017:2450401.https://doi.org/10.1155/2017/2450401.

28. Matusiak L, Szczech J, Bieniek A, Nowicka-Suszko D, Szepietowski JC. Increased interleukin (IL)-17 serum levels in patients with hidradenitis suppurativa: implications for treatment with anti-IL-17 agents. J Am Acad Dermatol. 2017;76:670–5. https://doi.org/10.1016/j.jaad.2016.10.042.

29. Matusiak L, Bieniek A, Szepietowski JC. Increased serum tumour necrosis factor-alpha in hidradenitis suppurativa patients: is there a basis for treatment with anti-tumour necrosis factor-alpha agents? Acta Derm Venereol. 2009;89(6):601–3.

30. Hessam S, Sand M, Gambichler T, Bechara FG. Correlation of inflammatory serum markers with disease severity in patients with hidradenitis suppurativa (HS). J Am Acad Dermatol. 2015;73:998–1005. https://doi.org/10.1016/j.jaad.2015.08.052.

31. Ring HC, Bay L, Nilsson M, Kallenbach K, Miller IM, Saunte DM, et al. Bacterial biofilm in chronic lesions of hidradenitis suppurativa. Br J Dermatol. 2017;176:993–1000. https://doi.org/10.1111/bjd.15007.

32. Guet-Revillet H, Jais JP, Ungeheuer MN, Coignard-Biehler H, Duchatelet S, Delage M, et al. The microbiological landscape of anaerobic infections in hidradenitis suppurativa: a prospective metagenomic study. Clin Infect Dis. 2017;65:282–91. https://doi.org/10.1093/cid/cix285.

33. Nikolakis G, Liakou AI, Bonovas S, Seltmann H, Bonitsis N, Join-Lambert O, et al. Bacterial colonization in hidradenitis suppurativa/acne inversa: a cross sectional study of 50 patients and review of the literature. Acta Derm Venereol. 2017;97:493–8. https://doi.org/10.2340/00015555-2591.

34. König A, Lehmann C, Rompel R, Happle R. Cigarette smoking as a triggering factor of hidradenitis suppurativa. Dermatology. 1999;198:261–4.

35. Sartorius K, Emtestam L, Jemec GBE, Lapins J. Objective scoring of hidradenitis suppurativa reflecting the role of tobacco smoking and obesity. Br J Dermatol. 2009;161:831–9.

36. Wiltz O, Schoetz DJ Jr, Murray JJ, Roberts PL, Coller JA, Veidenheimer MC. Perianal hidradenitis suppurativa. The Lahey Clinic experience. Dis Colon Rectum. 1990;33:731–4.

37. Freiman A, Bird G, Metelitsa AI, Barankin B, Lauzon GJ. Cutaneous effects of smoking. J Cutan Med Surg. 2004;8:415–23.

38. Bianchi L, Caposiena Caro RD, Ganzetti G, Molinelli E, Dini V, Oranges T, Romanelli M, Fabbrocini G, Monfrecola G, Napolitano M, Egan CG, Musumeci ML, Lacarrubba F, Micali G, Passoni E, Calzavara-Pinton PG, Venturini M, Zanca A, Offidani AM. Sex-related differences of clinical features in hidradenitis suppurativa: analysis of an Italian-based cohort. Clin Exp Dermatol. 2019;44:e177–80. https://doi.org/10.1111/ced.13861.. [Epub ahead of print]

39. Alikhan A, Lynch PJ, Eisen DB. Hidradenitis suppurativa: a comprehensive review. J Am Acad Dermatol. 2009;60:539–61.

40. Kohorst JJ, Kimball AB, Davis MD. Systemic associations of hidradenitis suppurativa. J Am Acad Dermatol. 2015;73(5 Suppl 1):S27–35.

41. Nazary M, van der Zee HH, Prens EP, Folkerts G, Boer J. Pathogenesis and pharmacotherapy of Hidradenitis suppurativa. Eur J Pharmacol. 2011;672(1-3):1–8.

42. Romaní J, Agut-Busquet E, Corbacho M, Herrerías-Moreno J, Luelmo J. Body fat composition in hidradenitis suppurativa: a hospital-based cross-sectional study. Int J Dermatol. 2017;56(3):e62–3.

43. Boer J, Nazary M, Riis PT. The role of mechanical stress in hidradenitis suppurativa. Dermatol Clin. 2016;34(1):37–43.

44. Jemec GB. Clinical practice. Hidradenitis suppurativa. N Engl J Med. 2012;366(2):158–64.

45. Harrison BJ, Read GF, Hughes LE. Endocrine basis for the clinical presentation of hidradenitis suppurativa. Br J Surg. 1988;75(10):972–5.

46. Mengesha YM, Holcombe TC, Hansen RC. Prepubertal hidradenitis suppurativa: two case reports and review of the literature. Pediatr Dermatol. 1999;16(4):292–6.

47. Jayasena CN, Comninos AN, Nijher GM, et al. Twice-daily subcutaneous injection of kisspeptin-54 does not abolish menstrual cyclicity in healthy female volunteers. J Clin Endocrinol Metab. 2013;98(11):4464–74.

48. Kromann CB, Deckers IE, Esmann S, Boer J, Prens EP, Jemec GB. Risk factors, clinical course and long-term prognosis in hidradenitis suppurativa: a cross-sectional study. Br J Dermatol. 2014;171(4):819–24.

49. Dessinioti C, Katsambas A, Antoniou C. Hidradenitis suppurrativa (acne inversa) as a systemic disease. Clin Dermatol. 2014;32(3):397–408.

50. Martorell A, Wortsman X, Alfageme F, Roustan G, Arias-Santiago S, Catalano O, Scotto di Santolo M, Zarchi K, Bouer M, Gaitini D, Gonzalez C, Bard R, García-Martínez FJ, Mandava A. Ultrasound evaluation as a complementary test in hidradenitis suppurativa: proposal of a standardized report. Dermatol Surg. 2017;43(8):1065–73.

51. Wortsman X, Moreno C, Soto R, Arellano J, et al. Ultrasound in-depth characterization and staging of hidradenitis suppurativa. Dermatol Surg. 2013;39:1835–42.

52. Martorell A, Segura Palacios JM. Ultrasound examination of hidradenitis suppurativa. Actas Dermosifiliogr. 2015;106(Suppl 1):49–59.

53. Lipsker D, Severac F, Freysz M, Sauleau E, Boer J, Emtestam L, Matusiak Ł, Prens E, Velter C, Lenormand C, Meyer N, Jemec GB. The ABC of hidradenitis suppurativa: a validated glossary on how to name lesions. Dermatology. 2016;232(2):137–42.

54. Revuz J. Hidradenitis suppurativa. J Eur Acad Dermatol Venereol. 2009;23(9):985–98.

55. Lipsker D, Revuz J. Phenotypic characterization of patients with hidradenitis suppurativa. Dermatology. 2016;232(4):521.

56. van der Zee HH, Jemec GB. New insights into the diagnosis of hidradenitis suppurativa: clinical presentations and phenotypes. J Am Acad Dermatol. 2015;73(5 Suppl 1):S23–6.

57. Zouboulis CC, Desai N, Emtestam L, Hunger RE, Ioannides D, Juhász I, Lapins J, Matusiak L, Prens EP, Revuz J, Schneider-Burrus S, Szepietowski JC, van der Zee HH, Jemec GB. European S1 guideline for the treatment of hidradenitis suppurativa/acne inversa. J Eur Acad Dermatol Venereol. 2015;29(4):619–44.

58. Hurley HJ. Axillary hyperhidrosis, apocrine bromhidrosis, hidradenitis suppurativa, and familial benign pemphigus: surgical approach. In: Roenigk RK, Roenigk HH, editors. Dermatologic surgery. New York: Marcel Dekker; 1989. p. 729–39.

59. Sartorius K, Lapins J, Emtestam L, Jemec GB. Suggestions for uniform outcome variables when reporting treatment effects in hidradenitis suppurativa. Br J Dermatol. 2003;149(1):211–3.

60. Amano M, Grant A, Kerdel FA. A prospective open-label clinical trial of adalimumab for the treatment of hidradenitis suppurativa. Int J Dermatol. 2010;49(8):950–5.

61. Chiricozzi A, Faleri S, Franceschini C, Caro RD, Chimenti S, Bianchi L. AISI: a new disease severity assessment tool for hidradenitis suppurativa. Wounds. 2015;27(10):258–64.

62. Kimball AB, Kerdel F, Adams D, Mrowietz U, Gelfand JM, Gniadecki R, Prens EP, Schlessinger J, Zouboulis CC, van der Zee HH, Rosenfeld M, Mulani P, Gu Y, Paulson S, Okun M, Jemec GB. Adalimumab for the treatment of moderate to severe Hidradenitis suppurativa: a parallel randomized trial. Ann Intern Med. 2012;157(12):846–55.

63. Zouboulis CC, Tzellos T, Kyrgidis A, Jemec GBE, Bechara FG, Giamarellos-Bourboulis EJ, Ingram JR, Kanni T, Karagiannidis I, Martorell A, Matusiak Ł, Pinter A, Prens EP, Presser D, Schneider-Burrus S, von Stebut E, Szepietowski JC, van der Zee HH, Wilden SM, Sabat R, European Hidradenitis Suppurativa Foundation Investigator Group. Development and validation of the International Hidradenitis Suppurativa Severity Score System (IHS4), a novel dynamic scoring system to assess HS severity. Br J Dermatol. 2017;177(5):1401–9.

64. Kimball AB, Jemec GB, Yang M, Kageleiry A, Signorovitch JE, Okun MM, Gu Y, Wang K, Mulani P, Sundaram M. Assessing the validity, responsiveness and meaningfulness of the Hidradenitis Suppurativa Clinical Response (HiSCR) as the clinical endpoint for hidradenitis suppurativa treatment. Br J Dermatol. 2014;171(6):1434–42.

65. Wortsman X, Castro A, Figueroa A. Color Doppler ultrasound assessment of morphology and types of fistulous tracts in hidradenitis suppurativa (HS). J Am Acad Dermatol. 2016;75(4):760–7.

66. Caposiena Caro RD, Solivetti FM, Bianchi L. Power Doppler ultrasound assessment of vascularization in hidradenitis suppurativa lesions. J Eur Acad Dermatol Venereol. 2018;32:1360–7.

67. Saunte DML, Jemec GBE. Hidradenitis suppurativa: advances in diagnosis and treatment. JAMA. 2017;318(20):2019–32.. Review.

68. Margesson LJ, Danby FW. Hidradenitis suppurativa. Best Pract Res Clin Obstet Gynaecol. 2014;28(7):1013–27.

69. Canoui-Poitrine F, Revuz JE, Wolkenstein P, et al. Clinical characteristics of a series of 302 French patients with hidradenitis suppurativa, with an analysis of factors associated with disease severity. J Am Acad Dermatol. 2009;61(1):51–7.

70. Simonart T. Hidradenitis suppurativa and smoking. J Am Acad Dermatol. 2010;62(1):149–50.

71. Danby FW, Margesson LJ. Hidradenitis suppurativa. Dermatol Clin. 2010;28(4):779–93.

72. Di Landro A, Cazzaniga S, Parazzini F, et al. Family history, body mass index, selected dietary factors, menstrual history, and risk of moderate to severe acne in adolescents and young adults. J Am Acad Dermatol. 2012;67(6):1129–35.

73. Caposiena Caro RD, Cannizzaro MV, Botti E, Di Raimondo C, Di Matteo E, Gaziano R, Bianchi L. Clindamycin versus clindamycin plus rifampicin in Hidradenitis Suppurativa treatment: clinical and ultrasound observations. J Am Acad Dermatol. 2019;80:1314–21.

74. Gulliver W, Zouboulis CC, Prens E, Jemec GB, Tzellos T. Evidence-based approach to the treatment of hidradenitis suppurativa/acne inversa, based on the European guidelines for hidradenitis suppurativa. Rev Endocr Metab Disord. 2016;17(3):343–51.. Review.

75. Zouboulis CC, Bechara FG, Dickinson-Blok JL, Gulliver W, Horváth B, Hughes R, Kimball AB, Kirby B, Martorell A, Podda M, Prens EP, Ring HC, Tzellos T, van der Zee HH, van Straalen KR, Vossen ARJV, Jemec GBE. Hidradenitis suppurativa/acne inversa: a practical framework for treatment optimization - systematic review and recommendations from the HS ALLIANCE working group. J Eur Acad Dermatol Venereol. 2019;33(1):19–31.

76. Rosi E, Pescitelli L, Ricceri F, Di Cesare A, Novelli A, Pimpinelli N, Prignano F. Clindamycin as unique antibiotic choice in Hidradenitis Suppurativa. Dermatol Ther. 2018;5:e12792.

77. Join-Lambert O, Coignard H, Jais JP, et al. Efficacy of rifampin-moxifloxacin-metronidazole combination therapy in hidradenitis suppurativa. Dermatology. 2011;222:49–58.

78. Join-Lambert O, Coignard-Biehler H, Jais JP, Delage M, Guet-Revillet H, Poirée S, Duchatelet S, Jullien V, Hovnanian A, Lortholary O, Nassif X, Nassif A. Efficacy of ertapenem in severe hidradenitis suppurativa: a pilot study in a cohort of 30 consecutive patients. J Antimicrob Chemother. 2016;71(2):513–20.

79. Braunberger TL, Nartker NT, Nicholson CL, Nahhas AF, Parks-Miller A, Hanna Z, Jayaprakash R, Ramesh MS, Rambhatla PV, Hamzavi IH. Ertapenem—a potent treatment for clinical and quality of life improvement in patients with hidradenitis suppurativa. Int J Dermatol. 2018;57(9):1088–93.

80. Mendes-Bastos P, Martorell A, Magina S. Ertapenem for the treatment of Hidradenitis suppurativa: how much do we need it? Actas Dermosifiliogr. 2018;109(7):582–3.

81. Chahine AA, Nahhas AF, Braunberger TL, Rambhatla PV, Hamzavi IH. Ertapenem rescue therapy in hidradenitis suppurativa. JAAD Case Rep. 2018;4(5):482–3.

82. Albrecht J, Baine PA, Ladizinski B, Jemec GB, Bigby M. Long-term clinical safety of clindamycin and rifampicin combination for the treatment of hidradenitis suppurativa. A critically appraised topic. Br J Dermatol. 2019;180:749–55.

83. Andersen RK, Jemec GB. Treatments for hidradenitis suppurativa. Clin Dermatol. 2017;35(2):218–24.

84. Kimball AB, Okun MM, Williams DA, Gottlieb AB, Papp KA, Zouboulis CC, Armstrong AW, Kerdel F, Gold MH, Forman SB, Korman NJ, Giamarellos-Bourboulis EJ, Crowley JJ, Lynde C, Reguiai Z, Prens EP, Alwawi E, Mostafa NM, Pinsky B, Sundaram M, Gu Y, Carlson DM, Jemec GB. Two phase 3 trials of adalimumab for hidradenitis suppurativa. N Engl J Med. 2016;375(5):422–34.

85. Zouboulis CC, Okun MM, Prens EP, Gniadecki R, Foley PA, Lynde C, Weisman J, Gu Y, Williams DA, Jemec GBE. Long-term adalimumab efficacy in patients with moderate-to-severe hidradenitis suppurativa/acne inversa: 3-year results of a phase 3 open-label extension study. J Am Acad Dermatol. 2019;80:60–69.e2.

86. Kimball AB, Sundaram M, Shields AL, Hudgens S, Okun M, Foley C, Ganguli A. Adalimumab alleviates skin pain in patients with moderate-to-severe hidradenitis suppurativa: secondary efficacy results from the PIONEER I and PIONEER II randomized controlled trials. J Am Acad Dermatol. 2018;79:1141–3.

87. Caposiena Caro RD, Cannizzaro MV, Di Raimondo C, Di Matteo E, Botti E, Rossi P, Bianchi L. Long-term efficacy and safety of adalimumab on a severe case of Hidradenitis Suppurativa. G Ital Dermatol Venereol. 2018; https://doi.org/10.23736/S0392-0488.18.06194-1.

88. Vossen ARJV, van Doorn MBA, van der Zee HH, Prens EP. Apremilast for moderate hidradenitis suppurativa: results of a randomized controlled trial. J Am Acad Dermatol. 2019;80(1):80–8. https://doi.org/10.1016/j.jaad.2018.06.046.. Epub 2018 Jul 3.

89. https://clinicaltrials.gov/ct2/results?cond=hidradenitis+suppurativa&Search=Apply&recrs=b&recrs=a&recrs=d&age_v=&gndr=&type=&rslt=&phase=1&phase=2

90. Boer J, van Gemert MJ. Long-term results of isotretinoin in the treatment of 68 patients with hidradenitis suppurativa. J Am Acad Dermatol. 1999;40(1):73–6.

91. Boer J, Nazary M. Long-term results of acitretin therapy for hidradenitis suppurativa. Is acne inversa also a misnomer? Br J Dermatol. 2011;164(1):170–5.

92. Soria A, Canoui-Poitrine F, Wolkenstein P, et al. Absence of efficacy of oral isotretinoin in hidradenitis suppurativa: a retrospective study based on patients' outcome assessment. Dermatology. 2009;218(2):134–5.

93. Danby FW. Night blindness, vitamin A deficiency, and isotretinoin psychotoxicity. Dermatol Online J. 2003;9(5):30.

94. Mortimer PS, Dawber RP, Gales MA, Moore RA. A double-blind controlled cross-over trial of cyproterone acetate in females with hidradenitis suppurativa. Br J Dermatol. 1986;115(3):263–8.

95. Joseph MA, Jayaseelan E, Ganapathi B, Stephen J. Hidradenitis suppurativa treated with finasteride. J Dermatolog Treat. 2005;16(2):75–8.

96. Lee A, Fischer G. A case series of 20 women with hidradenitis suppurativa treated with spironolactone. Australas J Dermatol. 2015;56(3):192–6.

Ultrasound of Pigmented Melanocytic Tumors

4

Gaston Roustan and Irene Salgüero

Melanocytic neoplasias are composed of a proliferation of abnormal melanocytes, cells derived from neural crest. They are located mostly in the basal layer of the epidermis and the hair follicles. Pigmentation due to melanin deposit is their most characteristic feature, although some of them such as amelanotic malignant melanoma or Spitz's nevus are rarely pigmented. In the beginning these cells are only present in the epidermis (junctional nevi) aggregated in "nests"; with time they go to the dermis (compound or intradermal nevi) and occasionally to the subcutaneous fat (this is most likely occurring in congenital lesions).

Diagnosis is made mostly by visual skin examination and epiluminescence microscopy or dermoscopy, although the latter only allows us to identify changes in the epidermis, the dermoepidermal junction, and the papillary dermis but not the full dermal thickness or the complete depth of the lesion. Confocal reflectance microscopy, another noninvasive imaging technique, has a resolution almost similar to conventional histology, but is depth limited (papillary dermis), expensive, and available in few dermatologic centers. Final diagnosis requires histopathological confirmation.

With the appearance of the high-frequency transducers (>20 MHz), there is an increase in the use of ultrasound (US) in the study of the morphologic features of skin tumors [1], delivering complementary data about the shape, the topographic location, the homogeneity, the borders, the relation with adjacent structures, the thickness, and the margins of the tumor (lateral or depth extension). All the above help us to improve the initial management and the follow-up of the melanocytic neoplasia [2].

We are going to review the clinical and sonographic characteristics of the benign and malignant melanocytic tumors.

4.1 Benign Melanocytic Tumors

Benign melanocytic nevus, usually called "moles," may be congenital or acquired.

Congenital melanocytic nevi are present at birth (around 1% infants) and they usually have a large size. We classified them as:

- Small-sized: <1.5 cm
- Medium-sized: 1.5–20 cm
- Giant: >20 cm

They are characterized by a brownish well-defined solitary macule, usually with hypertrophic hair follicles in the surface (Fig. 4.1). They usually appear in the trunk, although other sites may be involved. Histopathological studies

G. Roustan (✉) · I. Salgüero
Department of Dermatology, Hospital Universitario
Puerta de Hierro Majadahonda, Madrid, Spain

© Springer Nature Switzerland AG 2020
R. L. Bard (ed.), *Image Guided Dermatologic Treatments*,
https://doi.org/10.1007/978-3-030-29236-2_4

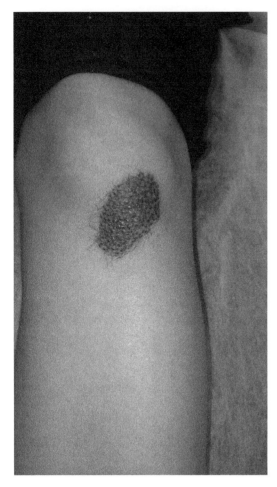

Fig. 4.1 Medium-sized congenital melanocytic nevus in the leg of a 7-year-old girl

reflect dense nevus cells reaching deep in the dermis and even subcutaneous tissue. Giant congenital nevi may be associated with leptomeningeal melanocytosis (neurocutaneous melanosis and increased but low risk (approximately 5%) of malignant transformation, especially if located in the axial line). They have a nonepidermal origin, so may begin as a dermo-hypodermic nodule.

US features of congenital melanocytic nevus are characterized by an increased wave-type epidermal thickness in the surface and a hypoechoic homogeneous, well-defined lesion of variable size presenting in almost all the dermis [1]. In the deep dermis, we may see a "cuff" around the hair follicle (Fig. 4.2). There is no increase in the vascularization (Fig. 4.3).

Acquired melanocytic nevi appear in the childhood or adolescence with sun exposure in the first years of life a predisposing factor and are more frequent in patients with fair skin (phototype I/II). They begin as a flat macular lesion (intraepidermal junctional nevus), with time cell nests extend to the superficial dermis and the lesions become more elevated (compound nevus) (Fig. 4.4), and finally almost all the nevi cells are present in the dermis, gradually loosing pigmentation (intradermal Miescher's and Unna's nevi). It is remarkable that melanoma associated with nevus (around 33% of all malignant melanomas) begins in the epidermal part of the nevus.

Fig. 4.2 Grayscale US congenital melanocytic nevus: dermal hypoechoic lesion with "cuffs" around hypertrophic follicles

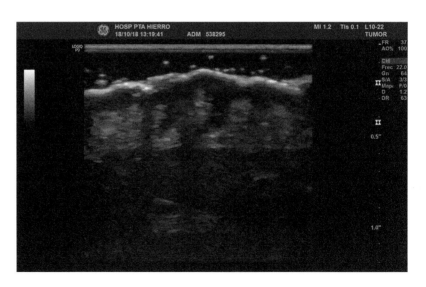

Fig. 4.3 Color Doppler congenital melanocytic nevus: absence of vascularization

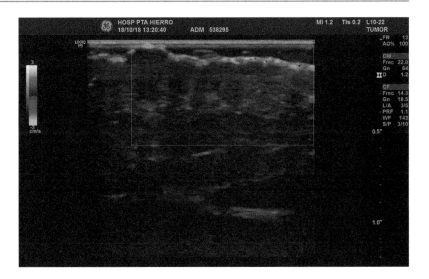

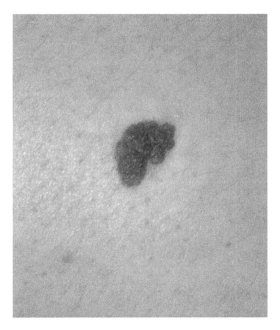

Fig. 4.4 Acquired melanocytic nevus in the trunk of a 25-year-old boy

Sonographic studies of common acquired nevi show the typical characteristics of a benign lesion: hypoechoic, well-delimited, homogenous lesion located in the upper dermis without increase in Doppler flow (Fig. 4.5a, b) [2]. Harland et al. [3] reported that melanocytic nevi are mainly hypoechoic with many small echoes, are symmetric, and usually are well delimited from the adjacent dermis. Similar features are also observed in dysplastic or atypical nevi, a variant with a high risk in the development of melanoma, especially in familiar atypical nevus syndrome.

Blue nevi are benign proliferation of dermal melanocytes. They derived from melanocytic cells that did not complete their migration from the neural crest to the epidermis during embryogenesis and settle in the dermis. It is characterized by the appearance in adulthood of a bluish-black macule or papule in the cephalic region (Fig. 4.6) and distal areas (hands, feet). The color is due to the Tyndall effect (the preferential absorption of long light wavelengths by dermal melanin inside melanocytes in the superficial and middermis and the scattering of shorter wavelengths, representing the blue end of the spectrum, by collagen bundles).

Ultrasound studies show a dermal, oval (some authors suggest the term "dish") shape, hypoechoic well-defined homogenous lesion without increased vascular flow (Fig. 4.7a, b) [1]. Samimi et al. [4] reported that sonography was more specific (94%) than clinical examination (77%) and dermoscopy (74%) in the diagnosis of blue skin lesions. The sonographic features contributing to the differential diagnosis were location of the lesion, shape of the lesion, homogeneity, and increased posterior echogenicity.

Spitz's nevus is characterized by a pink-flesh-colored papule or nodule arising on the face of children. It may also appear in the trunk and

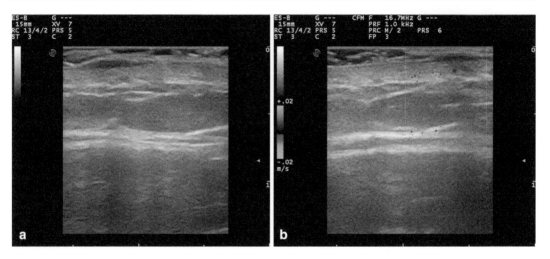

Fig. 4.5 (**a**) Grayscale US-acquired melanocytic nevus: superficial homogeneous well-defined hypoechoic lesion. (**b**) Color Doppler without increased vascularization

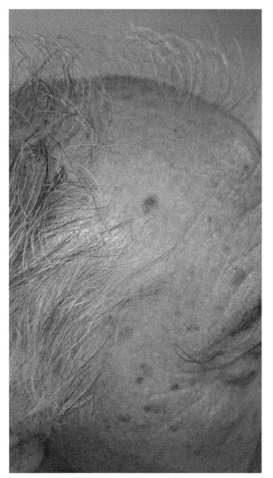

Fig. 4.6 Blue nevus in the face of a 70-year-old man

extremities (lower limb) (Fig. 4.8). There is a distinct hyperpigmented variant that appears as a small papule in the proximal part of extremities of young adults termed Reed's nevus. Histopathology may mimic malignant melanoma, with a proliferation in the superficial and middermis of epithelioid or fusicellular melanocytes (deep maturation).

There are very few descriptions of sonographic features of Spitz's nevus in the literature [1]. We may see a hypoechoic oval homogeneous lesion located in the superficial dermis (Fig. 4.9a), with a small increase in vascularization (Fig. 4.9b).

4.2 Malignant Melanoma

The incidence of skin malignant melanoma (MM) is increasing faster than any other cancer. Although less frequent than nonmelanoma skin cancer, it is responsible for the majority of the deaths attributable to cutaneous malignancies. Median age at diagnosis is 59 years. Risk factors for melanoma include: skin type, personal history of prior melanoma, multiple clinically atypical moles or dysplastic nevi, and a positive family history of melanoma. Predisposed patients subjected to environmental factors including excess sun exposure and UV tanning bed use are at greater risk.

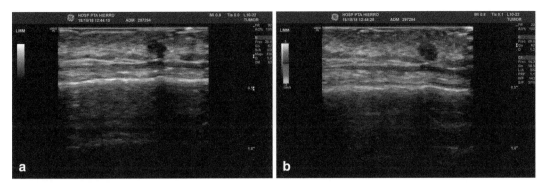

Fig. 4.7 (**a**) Grayscale US blue nevus: oval well-defined homogeneous hypoechoic in the middermis (courtesy Dr. Alfageme). (**b**) Color Doppler: no increase in blood flow (courtesy Dr. Alfageme)

Fig. 4.8 Spitz's nevus in the leg of an 11-year-old girl. Note two colors in the surface (red/brown)

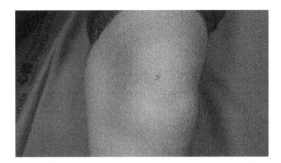

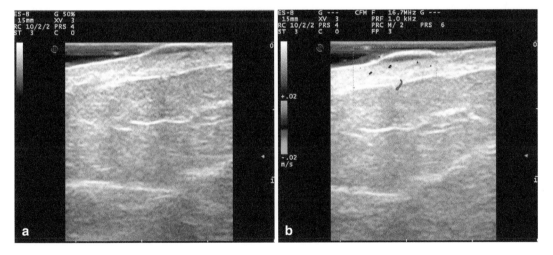

Fig. 4.9 (**a**) Grayscale US Spitz's nevus: similar characteristics than acquired common melanocytic nevus (courtesy Dr. Alfageme). (**b**) Color Doppler Spitz's nevus: slight blood flow increase in the bottom of the lesion (courtesy Dr. Alfageme)

There are four classic clinical MM variants: lentigo melanoma, superficial spreading melanoma (Fig. 4.10), acral melanoma (Fig. 4.11), and nodular melanoma. With the advent of targeted therapy and the potential therapeutic implications of the specific mutations among clinical subtypes of melanoma, we may differentiate between non-chronic sun damage-associated MM (BRAF mutation: superficial spreading melanoma, nodular melanoma), chronic sun-

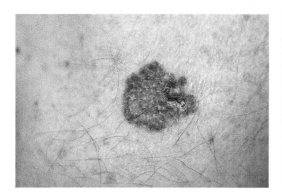

Fig. 4.10 Superficial spreading melanoma in the back of a 77-year-old man

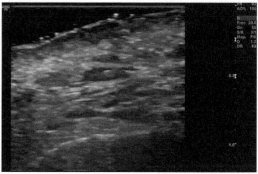

Fig. 4.12 Grayscale US lentigo melanoma in situ: superficial hypoechoic slightly irregular and inhomogeneous lesion that spreads along the epidermis

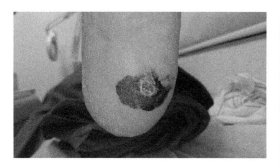

Fig. 4.11 Acral malignant melanoma in a sole of a 72-year-old man (excision: Breslow 5 mm)

induced damage MM (lentigo melanoma, solar elastosis, C-KIT mutation), and acral melanoma (palm, soles, nail; C-KIT mutation).

Histologic evaluation is the "gold standard" of MM diagnosis. Complete excision of the lesion is required for the histologic procedure if an MM is suspected. Once the diagnosis is confirmed, excision margins should be performed depending on tumor thickness (the most important prognostic factor). Clinical differentiation between benign and malignant melanocytic skin tumors is one of the most important issues in clinical dermatology.

Visual examination is still the most efficient procedure for clinical identification of cutaneous melanoma. The widely used acronym ABCDE (asymmetry, irregular borders, multiple variegated colors, diameter >6 mm, enlarging lesion) contains the primary clinical criteria for diagnosing suspected cutaneous MM. Sometimes the letter F (funny, ugly duckling sign) is added to the

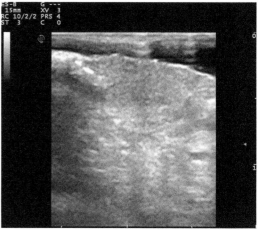

Fig. 4.13 Grayscale US acral malignant melanoma: hypoechoic V-shape lesion that reaches deep into the subcutaneous fat

classic acronym. The introduction of dermoscopy worldwide in the last decade increases diagnostic accuracy and sensitivity for melanoma and helps in the early detection of thinner tumors.

4.2.1 Primary cutaneous malignant melanoma

Harland et al. [3] made a complete sonographic description of malignant melanoma: homogeneous and hypoechoic dermoepidermal lesions (Fig. 4.12) rarely extending into the deep dermis or subcutaneous tissue (Fig. 4.13) as melanocytic nevi and frequently different in outline, having a "potato-shaped" appearance. Rallan et al. [5] remarked that surface heterogeneity is an important discriminator between melanoma and benign pigmented lesions. Melanomas generally are more attenuating than melanocytic nevi and have a higher surface heterogeneity and lower intralesional heterogeneity. The inhomogeneous structures (hyperechoic or anechoic) were correlated with rich intratumoral vascularization and fibrous stroma.

Malignant melanomas commonly show hypervascularity on Doppler examination (Fig. 4.14). Doppler techniques are used to assess the vascularization of skin tumors and the distribution and characteristics of intratumor vessels, thus increasing the diagnostic accuracy. Benign lesions do not show increase of vascularization (with some exceptions as glomus tumor), while malignant lesions are characterized by increase of flow peri- and intratumoral. Catalano et al. [6] stated that higher neovascularization vessel densities have an important risk of metastasis and worse prognosis. Botar Jid et al. [7] reported that the mean value of the Breslow index proved significantly higher whenever multiple pedicles were present compared to cases with a unique pedicle.

There are scattered reports describing the sonographic features of the different clinical variants of melanoma. Maldonado et al. [8] reported that lentigo melanoma, often found in the face of old people, is associated with marked solar elastosis reflected in a significant SLEB and high neovascularization (Fig. 4.15). Jaramillo et al. [9] described ungual melanoma as a solid, homogeneous, hypoechoic, ill-defined, hypervascular mass. Ill-defined/hypoechoic areas may present in the periphery related to peritumoral growth or infiltration. Silva-Feisner et al. [10] also observed that erosion of the boney cortex of the phalanx and the nail plate is a common feature.

Sonography is a reliable tool for evaluating the extent of the lesion and the determination of the involvement of adjacent structures and also for melanoma tumor thickness (ultrasound Breslow index) measurement for surgical planning preoperatively. Melanomas <1 mm have around a 99% 5-year survival, but melanomas

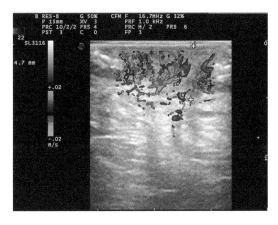

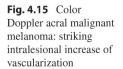

Fig. 4.14 Color Doppler lentigo melanoma: perilesional increase of flow

Fig. 4.15 Color Doppler acral malignant melanoma: striking intralesional increase of vascularization

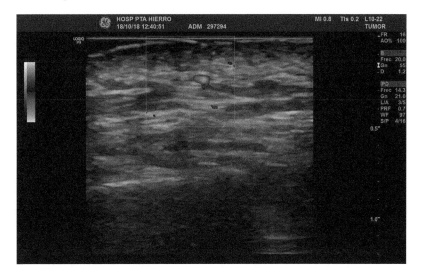

>4 mm reduce to less than 50% 5-year sur-
vival [11] . The tumor thickness of the majority
of thin melanomas is assessed correctly, although
in thicker melanomas associated with inflammation it could be more difficult [12]. In given cases,
the determination of the surgical margins is
supported by preoperative ultrasonographic
examination of the tumor thickness. Some
authors suggest sonographic depth measurement
may allow a one-step melanoma surgery [13].

Strain elastography (SE) also offers information about the relative elasticity or stiffness of the
tissues comparing the target lesion with surrounding normal tissues. Most malignancies show an
increase of stiffness versus benign neoplasia,
especially thicker tumors. Botar Jid et al. [7] also
showed that lesions with high elasticity proved to
have medium or low vascularization, while low
vascularization was observed in a higher number
of cases in lesions with medium elasticity.

Cutaneous melanoma metastases are an
important prognostic factor, and early recognition
may be very beneficial for patients to access to
new targeted therapies. Clinically they may be
solitary but are more frequently multiple, appearing as a rapidly growing bluish-red dermosubcu-
taneous papule or nodule, and may become
ulcerated with time. We should differentiate
between "satellitosis" (Fig. 4.16) (less than 5 cm

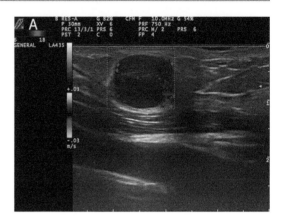

Fig. 4.17 Color Doppler: a well-defined oval homogenous hypoechoic lesion with peri- and intralesional
increase of vascularization

away from primary lesion, N2c or N3a if >4, stage
III AJCC 8th edition) and "in-transit metastases"
(more than 5 cm, N2c or N3a if >4, stage III AJCC
8th edition) and "cutaneous metastases" (far from
locoregional lymph node, M1a, stage IV AJCC
8th edition).

Sonography is a perfect tool for early detection of melanoma metastases. They present as
oval, regular, hypoechoic homogeneous lesions,
with very low internal echoes, showing necrotic
areas with anechoic appearance, and rarely an
irregular or polycyclic shape showing a perilesional and/or intralesional pattern on Doppler
examination (Fig. 4.17).

Solivetti [13] considered that US examination
with high-frequency probes is the best diagnostic
choice for this kind of lesions, better than telethermography and even PET-CT, because the latter has no high spatial resolution and the minimal
detectable dimension of the lesion must be at
least 5 mm, although he pointed out that a prolonged execution time (not less than 30′–40′ for
each limb or body area) is needed and is dependent on the operator's skills.

4.2.2 Lymph node melanoma metastases

Another important aspect of US in melanoma
patients is lymph node involvement assessment
and follow-up. Currently many specialists are con-

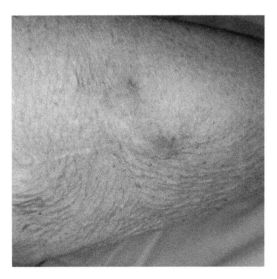

Fig. 4.16 Melanoma satellitosis near excision scar in an
82-year-old female patient

vinced, in view of the results of the latest clinical trials, that there is no survival benefit in performing total lymphadenectomy in patients with low-risk sentinel node metastasis (single node, intranodal/subcapsular, tumor load <1 mm). In these patients, a sonographic study every 4 months during the first 2 years and every 6 months until the fifth year is recommended. B mode assessment includes short-long (S:L) axis ratio, hilum, nodal border, echogenicity, intranodal necrosis, and ancillary features. Doppler assessment included distribution of vascularity, resistive index (RI), and pulsatility index (PI). Wortsman proposed a method for performing sonographic locoregional staging in melanoma [1]: start from primary lesion or scar, follow 10–20 cm around the primary region and study the entire extremity, follow the superficial vein tract and lymphatic drainage, and study ipsilateral and contralateral nodal stations (supra- and infraclavicular in case of head and neck melanoma).

Finally, promising new horizons in the use of US in melanoma patients have been recently reported. Bertelsen et al. [14] studied the feasibility of contrast-enhanced ultrasound (CEUS) for identification of SLN associated with cutaneous melanoma, using perflubutane, and concluded that this technique may be a useful adjunct technology in facilitating precise SLN dissection.

References

1. Wortsman X. Dermatologic ultrasound with clinical and histological correlations. 1st ed. New York: Springer Science; 2013.
2. Alfageme F, Roustan G. Ecografía en Dermatología y Dermoestética. 1st ed. Madrid: Ed. Panamericana; 2017.
3. Harland CC, Kale SG, Jackson P, Mortimer PS, Bamber JC. Differentiation of common benign pigmented skin lesions from melanoma by high-resolution ultrasound. Br J Dermatol. 2000;143(2):281–9.
4. Samimi M, Perrinaud A, Naouri M, Maruani A, Perrodeau E, Vaillant L, Machet L. High-resolution ultrasonography assists the differential diagnosis of blue naevi and cutaneous metastases of melanoma. Br J Dermatol. 2010;163(3):550–6. https://doi.org/10.1111/j.1365-2133.2010.09903.
5. Rallan D, Bush NL, Bamber JC, Harland CC. Quantitative discrimination of pigmented lesions using three-dimensional high-resolution ultrasound reflex transmission imaging. J Invest Dermatol. 2007;127(1):189–95.
6. Catalano O, Siani A. Cutaneous melanoma: role of ultrasound in the assessment of locoregional spread. Curr Probl Diagn Radiol. 2010;39:30–6.
7. Botar Jid C, Bolboacă SD, Cosgarea R, Şenilă S, Rogojan L, Lenghel M, Vasilescu D, Dudea SM. Doppler ultrasound and strain elastography in the assessment of cutaneous melanoma: preliminary results. Med Ultrason. 2015;17(4):509–14. https://doi.org/10.11152/mu.2013.2066.174.
8. Maldonado Cid P, Alfageme Roldán F, Suárez Masa D. Utilidad de la ecografía cutánea para el diagnóstico y la monitorización de la respuesta terapéutica del melanoma tipo lentigo maligno. Piel. 2015;30:328–30.
9. Jaramillo FA, Quiasúa Mejı CA, Martínez Ordúz HM, González Ardila C. Nail unit ultrasound: a complete guide of the nail diseases. J Ultrasound. 2017;20:181–92.
10. Silva-Feisner M, Álvarez-Véliz S, Wortsman X. Amelanotic subungual melanoma mimicking telangiectatic granuloma: clinical, histologic, and radiologic correlations. Actas Dermosifiliogr. 2017;108(8):785–7. https://doi.org/10.1016/j.ad.2017.03.008.
11. Crişan D, Florin Badea A, Crişan M, Rastian I, Gheuca Solovastru L, Badea R. Integrative analysis of cutaneous skin tumours using ultrasono_gaphic criteria. Preliminary results. Med Ultrason. 2014;16(4):285–90.
12. Fernández Canedo I, Moreno Ramírez D, Valdés Solís P, De Troya Martín M. Ecografía aplicada al manejo del melanoma maligno cutáneo. Actas Dermo-Sifiliográficas. 2015;106(S1):10–20.
13. Solivetti FM, Desiderio F, Guerrisi A, Bonadies A, Maini CL, Di Filippo S, D'Orazi V, Sperduti I, Di Carlo A. HF ultrasound vs PET-CT and telethermography in the diagnosis of In-transit metastases from melanoma: a prospective study and review of the literature. J Exp Clin Cancer Res. 2014;33:96. https://doi.org/10.1186/s13046-014-0096.
14. Bertelsen C, King KG, Swanson M, Duddalwar V, Pepper JP. Contrast-enhanced ultrasound with perflubutane for sentinel lymph node mapping in cutaneous melanoma: a pilot study. Laryngoscope. 2019;129:1117–22.

Ultrasound Diagnosis of Non-melanoma Skin Cancer and Malignant Melanoma

Robert L. Bard and Ximena Wortsman

5.1 Introduction

Clinical diagnosis of skin cancer is usually accurate. However, there is anatomical data that is impossible to deduct by the naked-eye examination such as the depth of a tumor. Nowadays, ultrasound is an integral part of dermatologic clinical evaluation of skin cancer. The literature has demonstrated an excellent ultrasound-histological correlation of the tumoral depth. Furthermore, ultrasound-guided biopsies and treatments are usually cost effective and can reduce morbidity.

On the other hand, almost pathognomonic ultrasound signs have been reported in basal cell carcinoma, the most common type of skin cancer in human beings.

The depth of melanoma can be measured by ultrasound, which can provide a sonographic Breslow thickness that has shown very good correlation with the histological depth.

On color Doppler, the level of tumoral vascularity can also be detected and commonly correlates well with the neoplastic angiogenesis. Last but not least, ultrasound supports the detection of the satellite, in-transit, and nodal locoregional metastases, which is relevant for melanomas.

5.1.1 Common Types of Skin Cancer

Skin cancer can be divided into non-melanoma and melanoma. The most common types of non-melanoma skin cancer are basal cell carcinoma and squamous cell carcinoma. Of them, non-melanoma tumors are much more frequent than melanoma. Furthermore, basal cell carcinoma is the most common type of skin cancer in human beings. Melanoma is less common but the most lethal one.

5.2 Basal Cell Carcinoma (BCC)

85% of BCC develops in the head and neck, in sun-exposed areas, and shows a preference for the thin skin of the face, such as the nose, lips, and eyelids.

The current shape of the ultrasound probes allows evaluating well all the locations including the ear pinna and nasal lesions.

While most BCC lesions appear on ultrasonography as well defined, mostly oval hypoechoic

R. L. Bard (✉)
Director, The AngioFoundation, New York, NY, USA
e-mail: rbard@cancerscan.com;
www.angiofoundation.org

X. Wortsman
Institute for Diagnostic Imaging and Research
of the Skin and Soft Tissues-IDIEP, Santiago, Chile

Department of Dermatology, Universidad de Chile,
Santiago, Chile

Department of Dermatology, Pontificia Universidad
Catolica de Chile, Santiago, Chile

© Springer Nature Switzerland AG 2020
R. L. Bard (ed.), *Image Guided Dermatologic Treatments*,
https://doi.org/10.1007/978-3-030-29236-2_5

masses, the majority of them show a variable number of hyperechoic spots. A higher number of hyperechoic spots have been reported to correlate well with the most aggressive forms such as morpheaform, or micronodular subtypes of BCC [1–5]. Identification of these foci is useful since neovascularity is less than that in other cancers (Figs. 5.1, 5.2, 5.3, and 5.4).

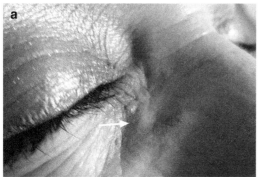

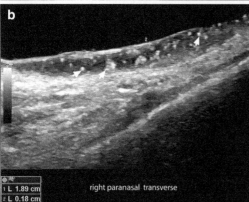

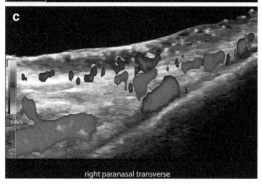

Fig. 5.1 Basal cell carcinoma of high risk. (**a**) Clinical image. (**b**, **c**) Grayscale and color Doppler ultrasound shows hypoechoic dermal band with more than seven hyperechoic spots (arrows) within the lesion (histology: morpheaform). Color Doppler shows increased vascularity within lesion [3]

5.3 Squamous Cell Carcinoma (SCC)

SCC is less common than BCC and also affects the sun-exposed regions. These tumors present as a hypoechoic lesion with irregular borders. Since the thickness or depth of invasion is an important predictor of metastases, the lesion should be followed along its entire course and as wide a perimeter as possible up to a draining nodal basin. Extra care is taken to find locoregional metastases and sonography of the liver and regional nodes may be performed simultaneously. The vascular pattern is diffusely increased throughout the entire mass as opposed to BCC where the neovascularity is less prominent and often at the bottom of the lesion. Due to the possibility of widespread penetration, vascular mapping for the main afferent vessels with 2D or 3D sonography is useful (Fig. 5.5).

5.4 Uncommon Dermatologic Malignancies

Dermatofibrosarcoma protuberans (DFSP) demonstrates a mixed pattern, usually with an ill-defined hypoechoic most superficial dermal and hypodermal part and hyperechogenicity with lobulated margins of the hypodermis (Figs. 5.6 and 5.7).

Merkel cell carcinoma presents as an ill-defined hypoechoic dermal and hypodermal focal area that usually demonstrates neovascularity (Fig. 5.8). Of interest, this lesion and its metastases tend to be radiosensitive and may be treated with external beam therapy if surgery is not possible.

Cutaneous lymphomas varieties have mixed echo patterns (the echo-poor ones may be mistaken for fluid collections) and variable vascularity. *Sarcomas* are hypoechoic except in the myxoid types or in the presence of internal necrosis and hemorrhage which may show an echogenicity with variable content of echoes and septa.

One of the main advantages of ultrasonography is the observation of the skin and deeper layers

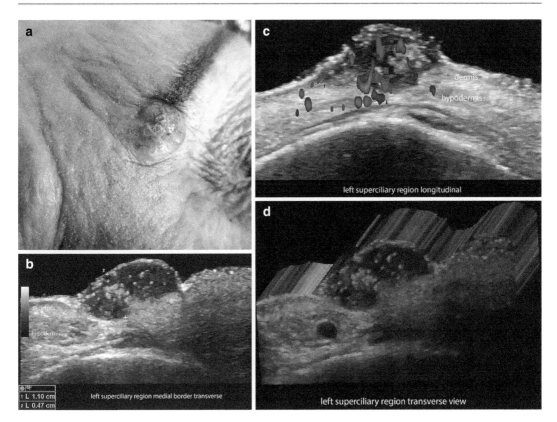

Fig. 5.2 Mixed high-risk and low-risk basal cell carcinoma. (**a**) Clinical image. (**b, c**) Grayscale and color Doppler. (**d**) 3D reconstruction ultrasound. Mixed subtypes shown in this lesion are micronodular (high risk of recurrence) and nodular (low risk of recurrence). The high-risk subtype appears as areas with a higher concentration of hyperechoic spots. Color Doppler shows hypervascularity in the periphery and within the lesion [3]

such as the fascia and the muscles. In deeper masses, MRI may be used to verify nonpenetration and integrity of the adjacent fascial plane.

5.5 Staging of Non-melanoma Skin Cancer

Sonography accurately measures the primary tumor dimensions in all axes and detects the blood flow within and adjacent to the lesion as well as the presence of deep layer involvement including nonpalpable metastases in deeper regional locations.

The satellite lesions are the metastases located at ≤2 cm from the primary tumor. The in-transit metastases are the ones located at >2 cm from the primary tumor.

Malignant ultrasound features of lymph nodes include the presence of eccentric or nodular thickening of the cortex, hypoechoic nodules in the medulla, a size of a lymph node ≥1 cm in transverse axis, and irregular or cortical hypervascularity.

This staging addition streamlines Mohs surgery and possibly provides one-phase treatment decreasing the recurrence rate and improving cosmetic outcomes.

5.5.1 Malignant Melanoma (MM)

Clinical diagnosis of MM is 54% accurate by histology and 20% accurate by non-microscopic nonspectral modalities. Solar lentigines situated in the upper epidermis are differentiated from

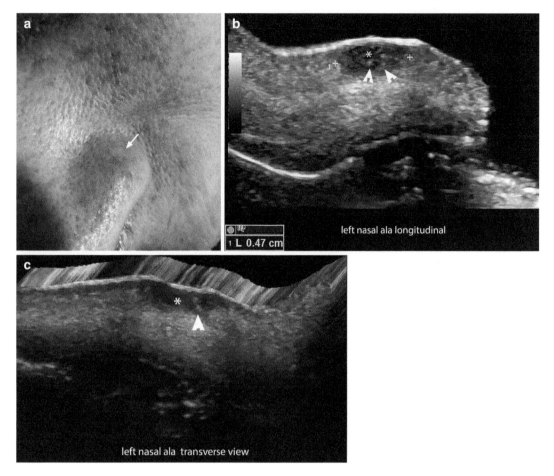

Fig. 5.3 (**a**) Clinical image nose (**b**) sonogram left nose. Clinical image. Grayscale. (**c**) 3D reconstruction. Transverse view of left nasal ala demonstrates well-defined hypoechoic lesion (asterisk) suggestive of low-risk subtype (histology: nodular subtype). Notice the small number of hyperechoic spots (arrowheads) within the lesion [3]

melasma and Becker's nevi located in the lower epidermis. Many benign pigmented lesions are removed preventively although there is only one melanoma found per every 33,000 nevi. Ultrasound screening is highly accurate for measuring melanomas ≥0.8–1 mm of depth. Dermoscopy, reflectance confocal microscopy (RCM), and other optical technologies such as hyperspectral imaging are complementary. Pathologists preview clinical pictures of a suspect lesion before they finalize readings due to inherent variability in interpretation. The finding of a subclinical metastatic focus near the lesion provided by newer ultrasound and spectral technologies facilitates histologic interpretation.

Planning optimal aesthetic conservation treatments requires advance knowledge of lesion borders, volume, and depth from the skin surface as well as adjacent vascular structures.

5.5.2　Ultrasound Findings of Primary Cutaneous Malignant Melanoma

Primary melanoma usually appears as a well-defined fusiform hypoechoic lesion. At frequencies below 14 MHz, it may appear echo free in a similar fashion to lymphoma due to densely packed homogeneous cell architecture (Fig. 5.9).

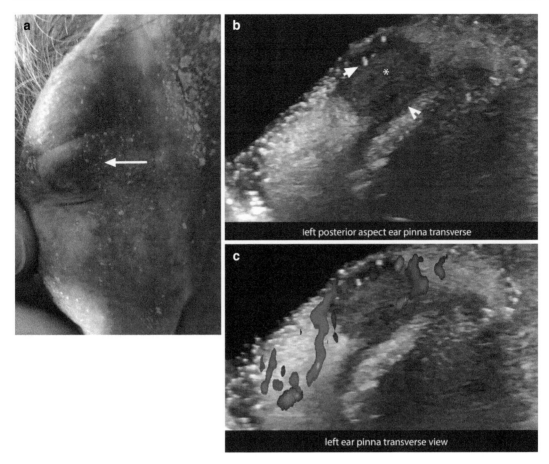

Fig. 5.4 Basal cell carcinomas of low risk that involve the auricular cartilage. (**a**) Clinical image. (**b, c**) Grayscale and color Doppler ultrasound (left ear pinna) shows round hypoechoic dermal structure (asterisk) that involves the surface of the auricular cartilage (arrowheads). Few hyperechoic spots (arrow) are detected. Slight increase in peripheral vascularity: histology; nodular subtype [3]

Melanomas that measure less than 0.4 mm can give a false-negative ultrasound exam while peritumoral inflammatory infiltrates may falsely increase the size of the tumor [6, 7]. On color Doppler, melanomas commonly appear hypervascular due to their prominent angiogenesis [8–11].

To date, contrast-enhanced ultrasound is not frequently used in the study of melanoma. Nevertheless, the assessment of angiogenesis has been reported to correlate well with the metastatic potential of melanomas [12–14].

Warts may also present a fusiform hypoechoic structure, but the flow tends to be more centrally located or in the sublesional region. Additionally, warts are commonly accompanied by thickening and irregularities of the epidermis due to the hyperkeratosis [15–17]. Although histogram vessel density analysis has not been reported in the dermatologic literature, it is widely used in the evaluation of primary endometrial, breast, and native prostate tumors [18] with good contrast-enhanced MRI correlation. PET/CT is usually the modality of choice to detect melanoma metastases; however, this technique may show false positives such as inflammatory processes or forgotten or displaced cosmetic fillers, and false negatives frequently in metastases that measure <5 mm. PET-CT imaging of metastatic disease is covered in a later chapter (Fig. 5.10).

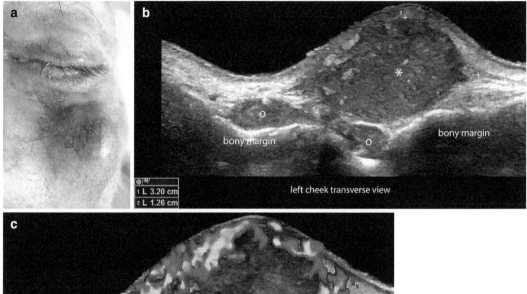

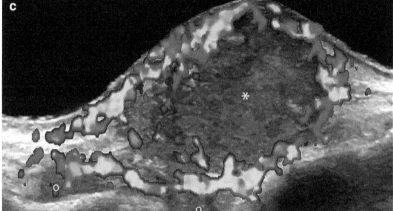

Fig. 5.5 (**a**) Clinical image. (**b**, sonogram **c**) Doppler sonogram. Grayscale and color Doppler ultrasound (left cheek) shows ill-defined, oval-shaped hypoechoic dermal and subdermal solid mass (asterisk) that involves the zygomaticus muscles and presents two well-defined, oval satellite lesions (0) which involve the bony margin and exit of the infraorbital nerve. On color Doppler there is prominent vascularity in the periphery and some vessels within the lesion (asterisk) [3]

5.6   Image-Guided Biopsy

New computer programs use nanotechnology and cybernetic modalities for image-guided biopsy and treatment options. Employing 3D Doppler sonography, the physician manually targets the area of highest tumor neovascularity. This is critical since only part of a mass may be cancerous and missed on nontargeted punch biopsies or superficial shave biopsies. The fusion of MRI with ultrasound permits image-guided biopsies sparing adjacent neurovascular bundles allowing customized ultrasound biopsies performed under local anesthesia.

5.7   Sentinal Lymph Node Biopsy (SNLB)

Ultrasound can guide the biopsy of regional nodal lymph nodes. Current guidelines suggest that a tumoral thickness greater than 0.8 mm reinforces the performance of a sentinel node procedure [19].

2D images and 3D reconstructions can document depth penetration and fascial invasion.

Ultrasound-guided biopsies of the tumoral regions with greatest architectural distortion and avoidance of thick vessels or areas with liquefaction or necrosis are clinically useful. An ultrasound-guided procedure may be required

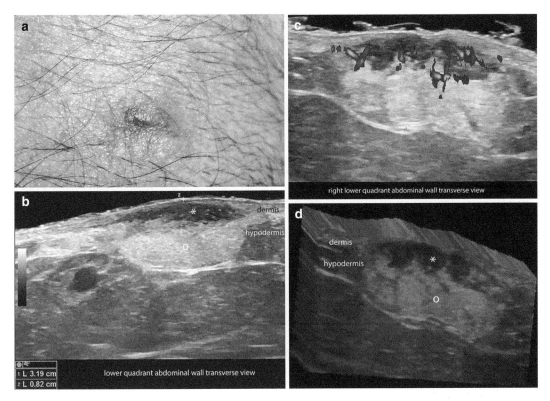

Fig. 5.6 Dermatofibrosarcoma protuberans. (**a**) Clinical image of right lower quadrant in a lesion that simulated a keloid. (**b**, **c**) Grayscale and power Doppler. (**d**) 3D reconstruction demonstrates upper hypoechogenicity (asterisk) and deeper hyperechogenicity (o) of the hypodermal part. Increased vascularity predominates in the upper part [3]

since 20% of the patients have been described to show nodal involvement [20, 21] (Fig 5.11).

5.8 Image-Guided Treatment Applications

3D Doppler ultrasound with dynamic contrast-enhanced-MRI (DCE-MRI) is the gold standard by which cancers are initially diagnosed and serially followed after treatment. The percentage of malignant vessels is quantified and re-evaluated in the identical tumor volume as serial follow-ups to the standard treatments using radiation, surgery, hormones, chemotherapy, cryotherapy, watchful waiting, and nonstandard treatments:

ablation using focal laser, focal ultrasound, photodynamic, radiofrequency, and microwave technologies. Vessel mapping allows the use of embolic treatments and immediate cessation of arterial flow appears as a surrogate endpoint to successful embolization. Ultrasound-guided FNAC identified 65% of all nodal metastases [22, 23]. Post-negative biopsy lymphoceles may be distinguished from recurrence and drained at the time of imaging [24].

Immediate cytologic confirmation of tumor permits withdrawal of the biopsy needle and insertion of a laser fiber, light source device, or cryogenic probe to treat and avoid seeding the biopsy site immediately. Thermocouple sensors prevent overheating of the adjacent nerves and

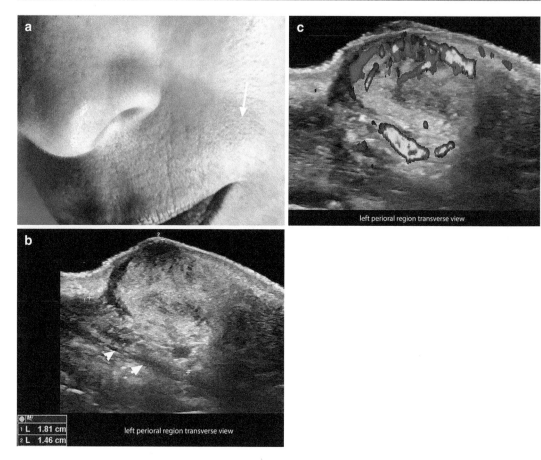

Fig. 5.7 Dermatofibrosarcoma protuberans. (**a**) Clinical image of perioral region. (**b**, **c**) Grayscale and color Doppler ultrasound demonstrates ill-defined oval-shaped, mixed echogenicity dermal and hypodermal mass with lower echogenicity in the upper part. There is infiltration of the left border of the orbicularis oris muscle (arrowheads). Color Doppler shows intense hypervascularity in the upper region [3]

sensitive tissues. Following ablation, the zone of destruction is confirmed with Doppler, contrast ultrasound, CT with contrast, or DCE-MRI. This outpatient procedure allows the patient to return to work immediately. Cutaneous melanoma with in-transit metastases has been successfully treated by laser technologies.

5.9   Comparison with Other Noninvasive Technologies

Multispectral imaging, OCT, RCM, and dermoscopy are limited by depth penetration, operator experience, availability, and diagnostic specificity [25]. Spectroscopy using electrical impedance, Raman analysis, and proteomic mass are newer procedures currently under study. Higher resolution technologies such as photoacoustic imaging and multiphoton analysis used in research laboratories are not clinically available yet promise unparalleled imaging of the epidermal layers and tumor vessel oxygenation measurements. While these technologies are covered elsewhere in the text more fully, the accuracy of sonography in the epidermis, dermis, and subcutaneous tissues is both operator and equipment dependent. Standard 2D linear sonograms at 40–100 MHz image the epi-

Fig. 5.8 Merkel cell carcinoma. (**a**) Clinical image. (**b, c**) Grayscale and color Doppler ultrasound shows oval-shaped hypoechoic nodule involving lower dermal border of the lateral aspect of the upper eyelid. Color Doppler shows intense blood flow in the lesion (arrow) and the periphery [3]

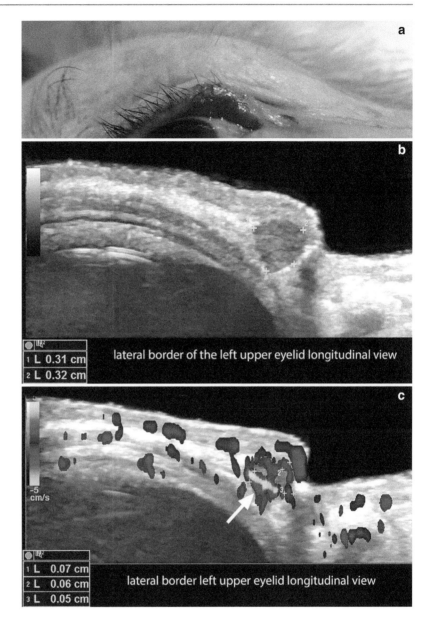

dermis. Probes using 15–22 MHz image the epidermis and dermis including the adjacent tissues 1–2 cm deep to the basal dermal layer. Real-time 3D probes at 16–24 MHz using broadband technologies provide high resolution of these structures to a 4–7 cm depth in seconds. Today's high-resolution equipment is widely available as an imaging technique.

5.10 Future Developments in Cancer Angiogenesis

Angiogenesis in the normal physiologic state is a new vessel formation in the areas of cellular reproduction, vessel development, and wound healing. Proangiogenic and antiangiogenic factors are balanced to control these functions.

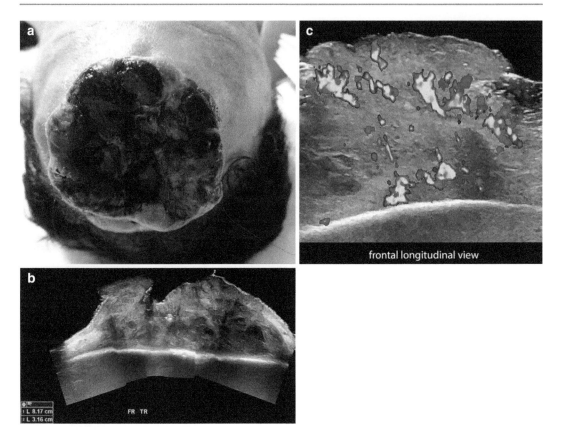

Fig. 5.9 Melanoma of scalp. (**a**) Clinical image. (**b**) Grayscale panoramic ultrasound. (**c**) Color Doppler ultrasound shows ill-defined hypoechoic mass extending into the musculoaponeurotic layer with increased blood flow [3]

Pathologic angiogenesis is the abnormal proliferation of blood vessels presumed to be stimulated by central hypoxia within the tumor. While vascular endothelial growth factor (VEGF) is the most important factor in the development of immature tumor vessels, it is not suitable as a clinical measurement in skin cancers.

Advances in ultrasound imaging include ultrahigh-frequency probes from 24 to 100 MHz providing image resolution up to 30 microns and ultrasound contrast agents allowing real-time imaging of tumor neovascularity. The technical aspects of Doppler flow detection with subharmonic imaging of microbubbles are covered in other articles.

Histopathology has demonstrated that tumors not only vary markedly over their surface volume in appearance but also have variations in microvasculature affecting aggression potential.

Tumoral immunohistochemical markers show strong correlation with tumor neovascularity with subharmonic contrast ultrasound [26].

3D ultrasound imaging quantifies vessel density in different quadrants improving targeting.

Contrast ultrasound imaging, now recently FDA approved for the skin, adds new dimensions in the serial assessment of treatment by monitoring quantitative changes in tumor vessel density.

Another potential usage of ultrasound is the provision of the depth and degree of vascularity of a superficial type of T-cell lymphoma such as mycosis fungoides that may allow electron beam therapy to be reduced from standard dose to low-dose modality [27].

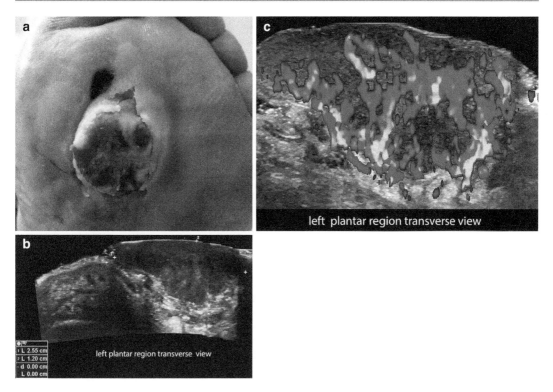

Fig. 5.10 Plantar melanoma, mostly amelanotic. (**a**) Clinical image. (**b**, **c**) Grayscale and color Doppler shows ill-defined hypoechoic mass extending into hypodermis with prominent intralesional neovascularity [3]

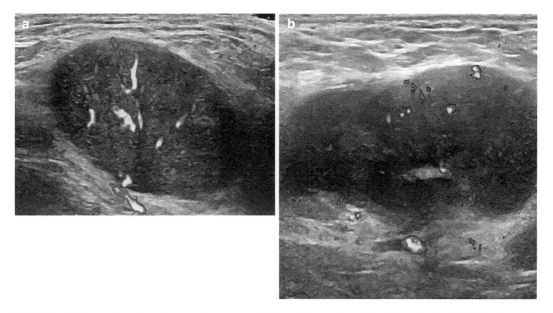

Fig. 5.11 Malignant lymph node vascular patterns. (**a**) Low degree of peripheral vascularity. (**b**) High degree of peripheral vascularity [3]

5.11 Sonography Changes Dermatologic Surgical Standards of Care

The American Institute of Ultrasound in Medicine (AIUM) has set forth standards of training for beginner, intermediate, and advanced uses of dermatologic ultrasound. While most high-resolution imaging is performed by radiologists and dermatologists trained in ultrasound, the shift to the point-of-care ultrasound (POCUS) usage has increased since the modality was first accepted by obstetricians. Contemporary examples are transrectal ultrasound biopsies by urologists and image-guided nerve blocks by anesthesiologists. The US Armed Forces train specialists in removing shrapnel or wooden fragments on the battlefield under ultrasound guidance. Plastic surgeons and aesthetic physicians prescreen patients for forgotten silicone deposits or unsuspected subdermal calcium before initiating cosmetic treatments.

Furthermore, in cosmetic fillers, the use of ultrasound may prevent serious complications such as blindness by direct vascular injection in feeding vessels of the ophthalmic artery. Therefore, imaging of skin cancers is a logical addition to the arsenal of skin cancer therapies.

On the other hand, the new noninvasive modalities working concomitantly with artificial intelligence (AI) may replace clinical recognition as a screening tool shortly [28].

Advanced photonics will lead to decreased biopsies due to improved margin recognition and earlier detection of tumor recurrence with modalities like in vivo multiphoton microscopy for basal cell tumors [29].

Reconstructive surgical success depends on skin viability and tissue perfusion. The preoperative and postoperative application of the dermal vascularity is another potential application of this technology.

Hyperspectral imaging has great potential with 100% specificity although a recent study showed a specificity of 36% [30]. The new technology of reflectance confocal microscopy is making great strides in burn diagnosis and

wound healing and is covered in a later chapter. However, confocal microscopy presents a very-low-depth penetration, usually less than 0.3 mm [31–38].

Thus, ultrasound remains the current first-choice imaging technique for studying skin cancer [39].

References

1. Lassau N, Spatz A, Avril MF, et al. Value of high frequency US for preoperative assessment of skin tumors. Radiographics. 1997;17:247–56.
2. Errico J, Pierre S, Pezet Y, et al. Ultrafast ultrasound localization microscopy for deep super-resolution vascular imaging. Nature. 2015;527:499–502.
3. Wortsman X. Atlas of dermatologic ultrasound. Cham: Springer; 2018.
4. Wortsman X. Sonography of facial cutaneous basal cell carcinoma. J Ultrasound Med. 2013;32:567–72.
5. Bobadilla F, Wortsman X, Munoz C, et al. Pre-surgical high resolution ultrasound of facial basal cell carcinoma: correlation with histology. Cancer Imaging. 2008;8:163–72.
6. Lassau N, Chami L, Chebil M, et al. Dynamic contrast enhanced ultrasonography and anti-angiogenic treatments. Discov Med. 2011;11:18–24.
7. Restreppo CS, Ocazionex D. Kaposi's sarcoma: imaging overview. Semin Ultrasound CT MR. 2011;32:456–69.
8. Tacke J, Haagen G, Horstein O, et al. Clinical relevance of sonographically derived tumour thickness in malignant melanoma. Br J Dermatol. 1995;132:209–14.
9. Guitera P, Li PX, Crotty K, et al. Melanoma histological Breslow thickness predicted by 75MHz sonography. Br J Dermatol. 2008;159:364–9.
10. Hoffman K, Jung J, el Gammal S, et al. Malignant melanoma in 20 MHz B-scan sonography. Dermatology. 1992;185:49–55.
11. Catalano O, Siani A. Cutaneous melanoma: role of ultrasound in the assessment of locoregional spread. Curr Probl Diagn Radiol. 2010;39:30–6.
12. Lassau N, Mercier S, Koscielny S, et al. Prognostic value of high frequency sonography and color Doppler for preoperative assessment of melanomas. Am J Roentgenol. 1999;172:457–61.
13. Lassau N, Koscielny S, Avril MF, et al. Prognostic value of angiogenesis evaluated by high frequency and Doppler ultrasound for preoperative assessment of melanomas. Am J Roentgenol. 2002;178:1547–51.
14. Lassau N, Spatz A, Avril MF, et al. Value of high frequency US for preoperative assessment of skin tumors. Radiographics. 1997;17:1559–65.
15. Nicolaidou E, Mikrova A, Antoniou C, et al. Advances in Merkel cell carcinoma pathogenesis and management. Br J Dermatol. 2012;166:16–21.

16. Pileri A Jr, Patrizi A, Agostinelli C, et al. Primary cutaneous lymphomas: a reprisal. Semin Diagn Pathol. 2011;28:214–33.

17. Galper SL, Smith BD, Wilson LD. Diagnosis and management of mycosis fungoides. Oncology (Willison Park). 2010;24:491–501.

18. Bard R. Advances in image guided oncologic treatment. J Targ Ther Cancer. 2016;1:52–6.

19. Music MM, Hertl K, Kadivec M, et al. Preoperative ultrasound with 15 MHz probe reliably differentiates between melanoma thicker and thinner than 1 mm. J Eur Acad Dermatol Venereol. 2010;24:1105–8.

20. Rossi CR, Mocellin S, Scagnet B, et al. The role of preoperative ultrasound in detecting lymph-node metastases before sentinel node biopsy in patients with melanoma. J Surg Oncol. 2003;83:80–4.

21. Van Rijk MC, Teertstra HJ, Peterse JL, et al. Ultrasonography and fine needle aspiration cytology in the preoperative evaluation of patients with melanoma eligible for sentinel node biopsy. Ann Surg Oncol. 2006;13:1511–6.

22. Ulrich J, van Akooi AC, Eggermont AM, et al. New developments in melanoma: utility of ultrasound imaging (initial staging). Expert Rev Anticancer Ther. 2011;11:1693–701.

23. Voit C, van Akooi AC, Schafer G, et al. Ultrasound morphology criteria predict metastatic disease of the sentinel nodes in patients with melanoma. J Clin Oncol. 2010;28:847–52.

24. Catalano O. Critical analysis of the ultrasound criteria for diagnosing lymph node metastases in patients with cutaneous melanoma. J Ultrasound Med. 2011;30:547–60.

25. Que SK, Grant-Kels JM, Longo C, et al. Basics of confocal microscopy and the complexity of diagnosing skin tumors. Dermatol Clin. 2016;34:367–75.

26. Gupta A, Forsberg M, Dulin K, et al. Comparing quantitative immunohistochemical markers of angiogenesis to contrast enhanced subharmonic imaging. J Ultrasound Med. 2016;35:1839–47.

27. Rivers C, Singh A. Total skin electron beam therapy for mycosis fungoides revisited with adjuvant systemic therapy. Clin Lymphoma Myeloma Leuk. 2019;19:83–8.

28. Glazer A, Rigel D, Winkelman R, et al. Clinical diagnosis of skin cancer. Derm Clinics. 2017;35:409–16.

29. Balu M, Zachary C, Harris R, et al. In vivo multiphoton microscopy of basal cell carcinoma. JAMA Dermatol. 2015;151(10):1068–74.

30. Hosking AM, Coakley B, Chang D, et al. Hyperspectral imaging in automated digital dermoscopy screening for melanoma. Lasers Surg Med. 2019;51(3):214–22.

31. Iftimia N, et al. Combined reflectance confocal microscopy/optical coherence tomography imaging for skin burn assessment. Biomed Opt Express. 2013;4(5):680–95.

32. Altintas AA, et al. To heal or not to heal: predictive value of in vivo reflectance-mode confocal microscopy in assessing healing course of human burn wounds. J Burn Care Res. 2009;30(6):1007–12.

33. Srivastava R, Reilly C, Francisco GM, Bhatti H, Rao BK. Life of a wound: serial documentation of wound healing after shave removal using reflectance confocal microscopy. J Drugs Dermatol. 2019;18(5):217–9.

34. Cameli N, Mariano M, Serio M, Ardigò M. Preliminary comparison of fractional laser with fractional laser plus radiofrequency for the treatment of acne scars and photoaging. Dermatol Surg. 2014;40(5):553–61.

35. Stumpp OF, Bedi VP, Wyatt D, Lac D, et al. In vivo confocal imaging of epidermal cell migration and dermal changes post nonablative fractional resurfacing: study of the wound healing process with corroborated histopathologic evidence. J Biomed Opt. 2009;14(2):024018.

36. Terhorst D, Maltusch A, Stockfleth E, Lange-Asschenfeldt S, et al. Reflectance confocal microscopy for the evaluation of acute epidermal wound healing. Wound Repair Regen. 2011;19(6):671–9.

37. Lange-Asschenfeldt S, Bob A, Terhorst D, Ulrich M, et al. Applicability of confocal laser scanning microscopy for evaluation and monitoring of cutaneous wound healing. J Biomed Opt. 2012;17(7):076016.

38. Rajadhyaksha M, Marghoob A, Rossi A, Halpern AC, Nehal KS. Reflectance confocal microscopy of skin in vivo: from bench to bedside. Lasers Surg Med. 2017;49(1):7–19.

39. Catalano O, Roldan F, Varelli C, Bard R, et al. Skin cancer: findings and role of high resolution ultrasound. J Ultrasound. 2019; https://doi.org/10.1007/s40477-019-00379-0.

Assessment of Efficacy of Systemic Therapy in Patients with Metastatic Melanoma

Philip Friedlander, William Simpson, and Cora Cajulis

It is estimated that in the United States in 2018, there were 91,270 new cases of melanoma diagnosed and 9320 melanoma-related deaths [1]. The American Joint Committee on Cancer version 8 staging system classifies melanoma into four stages [2]. Stages I and II include melanoma localized to the primary site and are determined by the depth of invasion (Breslow thickness) and the presence or absence of ulceration. Stage III melanoma includes metastasis to regional lymph nodes or the development of in-transit metastases along the regional dermal lymphatics. Stage IV melanoma is defined by the presence of distant metastases and is subdivided into four substages. Stage IV M1a includes spread to distant soft tissue or lymph nodes, M1b to the lungs, M1c to visceral sites other than the central nervous system, and M1d to the central nervous system.

Some patients with stage III melanoma present with macroscopic regional lymphadenopathy, while in others the lymph node involvement is identified through the performance of a sentinel

lymph node (SLN) biopsy [3]. With 10-year follow-up, 1347 patients with a primary melanoma with a Breslow thickness between 1.2 and 3.5 mm (intermediate thickness) were randomized to observation of the lymph node basin versus performance of a sentinel lymph node biopsy. Ten-year disease-free survival was significantly improved in the SLN group as compared to the observation group (71.3% versus 64.7%, respectively; $p = 0.01$). Identification of sentinel lymph nodes often utilizes filtered technetium-99m sulfur colloid administrated intradermally in separate injections around the primary lesion site. Several sets of planar views are then obtained, and then the patient's body is marked corresponding to the site of radioactive nodes noted on these image sets (Fig. 6.1).

Overall survival of patients with unresectable stage III or distantly metastatic melanoma depends on the efficacy of systemic therapy. Until 2011 no therapy conferring survival benefit was Food and Drug Administration (FDA) approved to treat stage IV melanoma. The two FDA-approved therapies were the cytotoxic chemotherapy dacarbazine and the cytokine high-dose-interleukin-2 (HD-IL-2). Dacarbazine treatment led to responses in 5–20% of patients with the responses being largely partial and not durable [4]. HD-IL-2 conferred a 16% response rate and 5% durable complete response rate [5]. Advances in understanding how the immune system modulates melanoma and how driver muta-

P. Friedlander (✉)
Division of Hematology and Medical Oncology, Tisch Cancer Institute, Icahn School of Medicine, Mount Sinai Hospital, New York, NY, USA
e-mail: philip.friedlander@mssm.edu

W. Simpson
Department of Radiology, The Mount Sinai Hospital, New York, NY, USA

Cora Cajulis
The Mount Sinai Hospital, New York, NY, USA

© Springer Nature Switzerland AG 2020
R. L. Bard (ed.), *Image Guided Dermatologic Treatments*,
https://doi.org/10.1007/978-3-030-29236-2_6

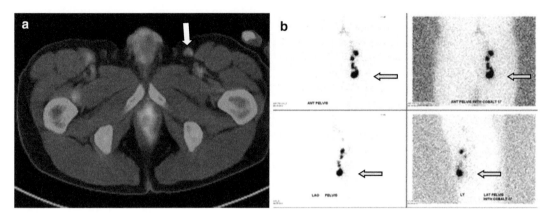

Fig. 6.1 Use of lymphoscintigraphy to map regional lymph nodes to which a primary melanoma drains. A 53-year-old male with subungual melanoma of the left great toe. Initial PET/CT (**a**) showed asymmetric FDG uptake with an SUVmax of 3.1 within a left inguinal lymph node with a preserved fatty hilum (white arrow). Since there was a preserved fatty hilum and relatively low SUV, the possibility of a reactive lymph node was consid-ered. As such, lymphoscintigraphy was performed with injection of Tc-99m sulfur colloid around the left great toe lesion. Imaging of the pelvis (**b**) revealed a sentinel lymph node (yellow arrow) with additional secondary echelon nodes in the left external iliac chain. Note the easier local-ization of the lymph nodes to the inguinal region with the use of the cobalt 57 mat that reveals a silhouette of the body (right-sided images in **b**)

tions in the BRAF signaling protein promote survival and proliferation have led in the past 10 years to FDA approval of immunotherapies tar-geting regulatory networks in the immune system and molecularly targeted therapies which block proliferative signaling through BRAF. Typically when assessing efficacy of a systemic therapy, imaging studies to assess interval change in metastatic burden are performed every couple of months. The advent of efficacious immunothera-pies has changed the paradigm that an increase in the size of a metastasis on imaging corresponds to tumor growth because an increase in tumor size may also reflect infiltration of immune cells into the tumor.

6.1 Immunotherapy

The activity of the immune system is tightly reg-ulated through the use of multiple positive and negative checkpoints. Activation of T-cells requires the T-cell receptor found on the T-cell membrane to bind to an MHC molecule com-plexed to an antigen-derived peptide sequence found on the membrane of an antigen-presenting cell. However additional costimulatory interac-tions are also necessary including the binding of CD28 present on the T-cell membrane to B7 pres-ent on the antigen-presenting cell membrane. Cytotoxic T-lymphocyte-associated protein 4 (CTLA-4) negatively regulates this costimulatory interaction inhibiting T-cell activity. Inhibition of CTLA-4 preserves T-cell activity and inhibits suppressor T-cells (Fig. 6.2). Ipilimumab is a fully human IgG1 monoclonal antibody that binds to CTLA-4 in an inhibitory fashion. To test the antitumor efficacy of ipilimumab, 676 patients with unresectable or stage IV melanoma were randomized in a 1:1:3 fashion to receive treatment with ipilimumab monotherapy, a pep-tide vaccine GP100, or both ipilimumab plus GP100. Median overall survival significantly improved following ipilimumab treatment being 10.1 months in ipilimumab-treated patients ver-sus 6.4 months in GP100-treated patients ($p = 0.003$) [6]. A pooled analysis of 12 phase II and III melanoma trials treating patients with ipi-limumab showed that the overall survival curve plateaus at 21% at approximately 3 years [7]. Ipilimumab was FDA approved in 2011 for the treatment of metastatic melanoma.

Programmed death-1 (PD-1) is another inhibi-tory checkpoint molecule expressed on the surface

Clinically Relevant Immune Checkpoints

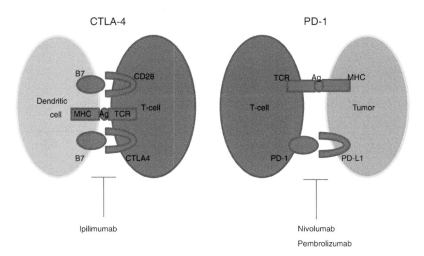

Fig. 6.2 Immune-mediated regulatory checkpoints. CTLA-4 and PD-1 negatively regulate immune activity by mechanisms as depicted on the left for CTLA-4 and right for PD-1. Ipilimumab binds to CTLA-4 in an inhibitory manner. Nivolumab and pembrolizumab bind to and inhibit the activity of PD-1

of T-cells. When PD-1 binds to its ligand PD-L1, T-cell activity is inhibited. Many melanomas select for the expression of PD-L1 leading to decreased T-cell activity in the tumor microenvironment (Fig. 6.2). Nivolumab and pembrolizumab are monoclonal antibodies that bind to PD-1 preventing binding to PD-L1. Both are FDA approved for the treatment of metastatic melanoma. The phase Ib KEYNOTE-001 study enrolled patients with metastatic melanoma to treatment with three different dosing schedules of pembrolizumab. Treatment with pembrolizumab conferred a 5-year overall survival rate of 41% in treatment-naive patients and 34% in the total patient population. Five-year progression-free survival was 29% in treatment-naive patients and 21% in the total patient population [8]. A multi-center randomized phase III trial assigned 834 unresectable melanoma patients to treatment with one of the two dosing regimens of pembrolizumab versus treatment with ipilimumab. Eligible patients had up to one prior systemic therapy. With 22.9-month follow-up, the median overall survival was 16 months for ipilimumab-treated patients but not reached in either pembrolizumab arm [9].This study supports the use of anti-PD-1 monotherapy prior to treatment with ipilimumab.

Nivolumab also inhibits PD-1 demonstrating efficacy in treating patients with unresectable melanoma. Phase I investigation demonstrated a 28% response rate in heavily pretreated melanoma patients with 26 of 94 patients developing a treatment response [10]. The CheckMate 037 study randomized 405 unresectable or stage IV melanoma patients in 2:1 fashion to treatment with nivolumab or chemotherapy. Treatment with nivolumab led to a higher and more durable rate of response, but no survival difference was appreciated [11, 12]. Lack of a survival difference may be the result of an increased dropout rate before treatment in chemotherapy-assigned patients. In fact the CheckMate 066 phase III trial enrolled 418 previously untreated BRAF wild-type advanced melanoma patients to treatment with nivolumab or dacarbazine chemotherapy demonstrating survival benefit from immunotherapy. Treatment with nivolumab conferred a significant overall survival benefit (HR 0.46, $p < 0.001$) with median overall survival of 37.7 and 11.2 months in nivolumab- and dacarbazine-treated patients, respectively [13]. Figure 6.3 shows an example of how CT and ^{18}F-FDG PET/CT can be used to determine response to treatment with anti-PD-1 monotherapy.

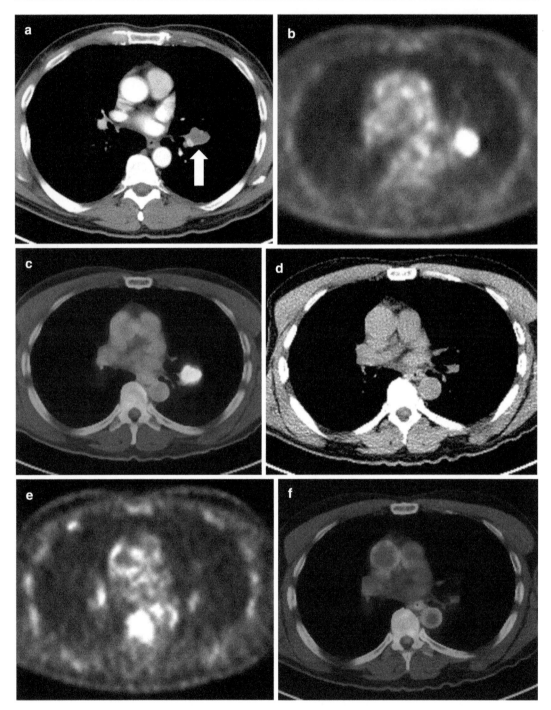

Fig. 6.3 Use of CT and¹⁸F-FDG PET/CT imaging to capture response of treatment with anti-PD-1 inhibitor monotherapy. A 62-year-old male with metastatic melanoma to the left hilar lymph nodes who progressed on ipilimumab treatment. PET/CT in May 2015 showed a 2.4 × 1.7 cm left hilar nodal mass on contrast-enhanced CT (arrow in **a**) which was FDG avid with an SUVmax of 8.7 on PET (**b**) and fused (**c**) imaging. He was then started on pembrolizumab. Repeat imaging in September 2016 shows that the left hilar mass has resolved. No mass is seen in the left hilar region on CT (**d**), and there is no longer FDG uptake on PET (**e**) or fused imaging (**f**)

Given the efficacy seen with CTLA-4 and PD-1 inhibitors and the difference of parts of the immune system targeted with these agents, the CheckMate 067 study was performed [14]. The study randomized 945 previously untreated unresectable or stage IV melanoma patients to treatment with nivolumab, ipilimumab, or combined therapy (ipilimumab concurrent with nivolumab). Treatment with nivolumab plus ipilimumab conferred a 58% response rate which was higher than the 45% and 19% response rates seen respectively following treatment with nivolumab or ipilimumab monotherapy. With a minimum 4-year follow-up, the median overall survival was not reached in the combination group, 36.9 months in the nivolumab group, and 19.9 months in the ipilimumab group. When deciding to treat a patient with anti-PD-1 monotherapy or dual-targeted therapy, the increased efficacy of concurrent CTLA-4 and PD-1 blockade needs to be weighed against relative high-grade immune-mediated toxicity risks (59%, 22%, and 28% rates, respectively, for ipilimumab- plus nivolumab-, nivolumab-, and ipilimumab-treated patients). Contrast-enhanced CT and ^{18}F-FDG PET/CT imaging can be used to assess treatment efficacy (Fig. 6.4).

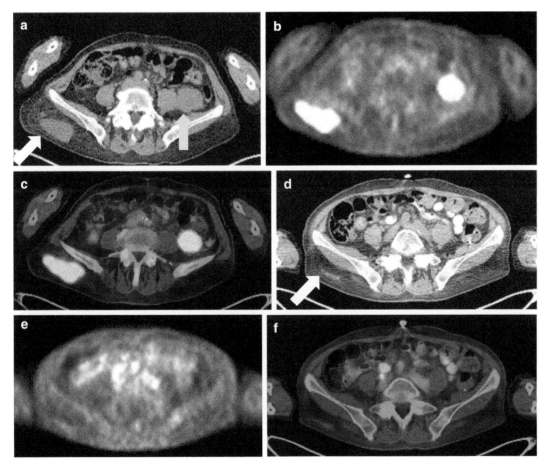

Fig. 6.4 Rapid response to treatment with nivolumab plus ipilimumab captured by ^{18}F-FDG PET/CT imaging. A 71-year-old female initially diagnosed with mucosal melanoma is found to have extensive metastatic disease within the chest, abdomen, pelvis, and bones. Pretreatment PET/CT showed a conglomerate mass in the right gluteal region measuring 7.4 × 3.4 cm (white arrow) and a 4.6 × 4.0 cm mass in the left retroperitoneum adjacent to the psoas muscle (yellow arrow) on non-contrast CT multiple other metastatic foci are not shown (**a**). Both lesions shown are FDG avid with an SUVmax of 16.7 in the right gluteal mass and SUVmax 17.3 in the left retroperitoneal mass on PET (**b**) and fused (**c**) images. Repeat imaging 2 months after only one dose of ipilimumab plus nivolumab showed marked response. The large right gluteal mass decreased to a thin linear streak (white arrow in **d**) on CT with no FDG avidity on PET (**e**) or fused (**f**) images. Similarly, the left retroperitoneal mass, and in fact all metastatic foci, disappeared with no residual FDG avidity

While inhibiting PD-1 or CTLA-4 provides clinical efficacy through modulating immune-mediated checkpoints, another immunotherapy strategy to treat unresectable melanoma patients is through the use of viral oncolytics. Talimogene laherparepvec (TVEC) is a herpes virus type-1 genetically modified to selectively replicate in tumor cells and secrete granulocyte-macrophage colony-stimulating factor (GM-CSF) [15]. The oncolytic virus is administered through intra-tumoral injection with the mechanism of action proposed through direct cytotoxic effects plus GM-CSF-mediated recruitment and activation of antigen-presenting cells. TVEC can be injected into dermal, subcutaneous, or lymph node metas-tases. Figure 6.5 characterizes small palpable subcutaneous nodules using ^{18}F-FDG PET/CT which were subsequently treated with intra-tumoral injection of TVEC leading to response.

The rate of durable response to TVEC treat-ment defined as an objective response lasting at least 6 months was assessed among 436 patients with melanoma containing an injectable lesion (cutaneous, subcutaneous, or nodal) and who did not have brain or bone metastases or more than three visceral metastases [16]. Patients were ran-domized to treatment with intra-lesional TVEC or subcutaneous GM-CSF. The overall response rate was 26.4% following TVEC treatment higher than the 5.7% conferred by subcutaneous GM-CSF. The rate of durable responses was significantly higher in TVEC-treated patients being 16.3% in the TVEC arm and 2.1% in the GM-CSF arm ($p < 0.001$). A case report of a 61-year-old woman with stage III melanoma with five in-transit metas-tases on the left leg treated with intra-lesional TVEC over a 6-month period with subsequent ^{18}F-FDG PET/CT demonstrates reduced or resolved activity in the injected lesions but the development of a new FDG-avid in-transit metastasis in the left thigh [17]. Therefore ^{18}F-FDG PET/CT imaging may be a good modality to monitor the efficacy of TVEC in patients with in-transit metastases.

6.2 BRAF-Targeted Therapy

The MAPK signaling pathway (Fig. 6.6) relays signals from activated cell surface receptors to RAS proteins leading to the dimerization and activation of A-, B-, and C-RAF proteins [18]. Active RAF activates MEK1 and MEK2, leading to ERK activation and cell proliferation. Activating mutations are present in approxi-mately 40% of melanomas [19]. More than 90% of the BRAF mutations are located at position 600 with the substitution of valine by a negatively charged glutamate (V600E BRAF mutation) leading to constitutive activation of BRAF [20].

Vemurafenib is a potent inhibitor of BRAF activity. In preclinical models, an analogue of vemurafenib inhibited the proliferation of V600E BRAF-expressing melanoma cell lines [21]. A phase I study evaluated the safety of oral vemu-rafenib in patients with advanced melanoma establishing efficacy in patients with melanoma containing V600E but not wild-type BRAF [22]. Rapid treatment responses were detected as evi-denced by decreases in metabolic activity of met-astatic deposits seen on ^{18}F-FDG PET/CT imaging performed 15 days after treatment initiation.

The randomized phase III BRIM-3 study treated previously untreated unresectable or stage IV patients whose melanoma contained a V600E or V600K mutation with vemurafenib or dacar-bazine chemotherapy [23, 24]. Treatment with vemurafenib conferred a significantly higher response rate of 48% compared to 5% for dacar-bazine. A significant improvement in both progression-free survival (PFS) and overall sur-vival was also seen with median PFS of 6.9 months following vemurafenib treatment as compared to 1.6 months following chemother-apy. Median overall survival increased from 9.7 months with dacarbazine to 13.6 months when treated with vemurafenib. Similarly the BRAF inhibitor dabrafenib conferred a 50% response rate and 5.1-month median PFS in V600 BRAF-mutated unresectable melanoma patients both significantly improved when compared to treatment with chemotherapy [25].

Treatment of patients with melanoma express-ing a V600 BRAF mutation with a BRAF inhibi-tor confers a high response rate but limited median PFS. Dual inhibition of the MAPK path-way through concomitant use of BRAF and MEK inhibitors has led to further increase in response rate and improvements in progression-free and overall survival. Treatment of V600-mutant

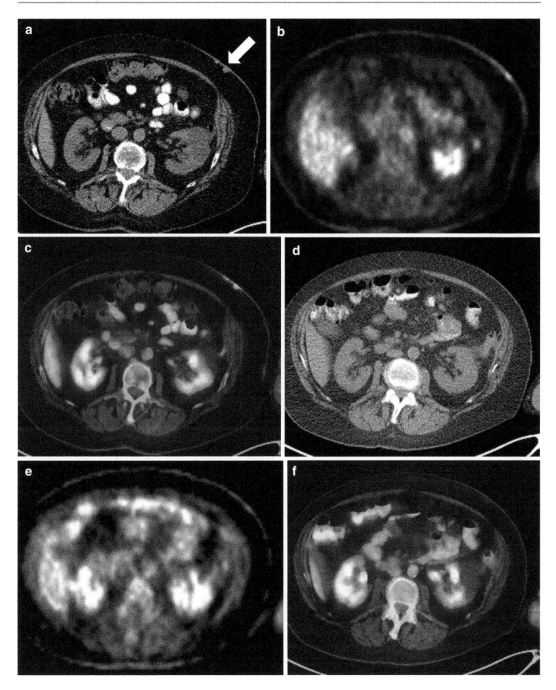

Fig. 6.5 Response to TVEC injections administered intra-tumorally into subcutaneous melanoma metastases. A 70-year-old female with small subcutaneous soft tissue nodules in the left anterior abdominal wall measuring up to 0.6 cm (arrow) on non-contrast CT (**a**). The nodules demonstrated FDG avidity on PET imaging (**b**) and fused image (**c**) with an SUVmax of 4.9. Patient was treated with TVEC injections into the subcutaneous nodules. Follow-up imaging 3 months later revealed near-complete resolution of the subcutaneous nodules with only slight skin thickening noted in the same area that was imperceptible on non-contrast CT (**d**) although there was residual mild FDG avidity on PET (**e**) and fused images (**f**) with SUVmax of 2.7

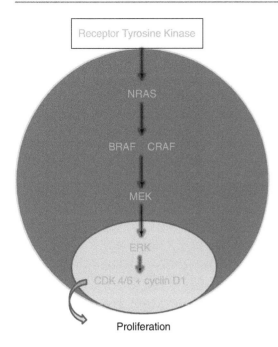

Fig. 6.6 Mitogen-activated protein kinase (MAPK) pathway. The pathway is activated in approximately 40% of melanoma through the selection of activating mutation in BRAF highlighted in bold. Targeted inhibition of BRAF and MEK leads to responses in approximately 70% of patients with melanoma containing a V600E BRAF mutation

BRAF melanoma patients with vemurafenib plus the MEK inhibitor cobimetinib conferred a 70% response rate and 12.3-month PFS both statistically significant when compared to the 50% response rate and 7.2-month median PFS following treatment with vemurafenib plus placebo [26]. Median overall survival also significantly improved from 17.4 to 22.3 months ($p = 0.005$). The Columbus phase III study randomized 577 melanoma patients with V600-mutated BRAF melanoma to treatment with the BRAF inhibitor monotherapy, either encorafenib or vemurafenib, or combined BRAF and MEK inhibition with encorafenib and binimetinib [27]. A significant improvement in median overall survival was seen in patients treated with dual-pathway inhibition as opposed to single-agent vemurafenib (33.6 versus 16.9 months; $p < 0.0001$).

A 3-year pooled analysis of clinical outcomes of unresectable V600 BRAF-mutated melanoma patients treated with dabrafenib plus the MEK inhibitor trametinib as part of two clinical trials that compared treatment to BRAF inhibitor monotherapy was performed showing 3-year PFS and overall survival rates of 23% and 44%, respectively [28]. Predictors for treatment progression were identified which included image-derived findings. Specifically patients with less than three organ sites involved, a normal serum lactate dehydrogenase level, and a sum of lesion diameters less than 66 mm were predicted to have better outcomes. The sum of lesion diameters was calculated using dimensions measured on contrast-enhanced CT imaging. Figure 6.7 demonstrates improvement in size and metabolic activity of melanoma metastases in a patient treated with dabrafenib plus trametinib.

6.3 Role of Imaging to Assess Treatment Efficacy

When treating a patient with advanced melanoma, efficacy is assessed by looking for change in the size and number of metastases through comparison of baseline imaging to interval on-treatment imaging studies. Identification of tumor progression through imaging allows for earlier discontinuation of ineffective therapy and initiation of alternative systemic therapy and decreases exposure to toxicity risk conferred by ineffective chemotherapy, immunotherapy, or targeted therapy. Typically interval change in tumor burden in stage IV melanoma patients undergoing treatment is reassessed at intervals of 2–3 months using modalities including but not limited to CT scans or fused ^{18}F-FDG PET/CT scans. With cytotoxic chemotherapy the identification of new metastases or the increase in size of prior metastases usually reflects tumor progression and leads to consideration of change in therapy. However this paradigm has changed with the advent of immune checkpoint treatment. When a lesion representing a metastasis is evaluated on a CT image, the lesion size can be measured, but the histologic makeup of the lesion is not readily apparent. Treatment with anti-PD-1 or anti-CTLA-4 antibodies can lead to immune cell infiltration of tumor. Therefore an increase in the size

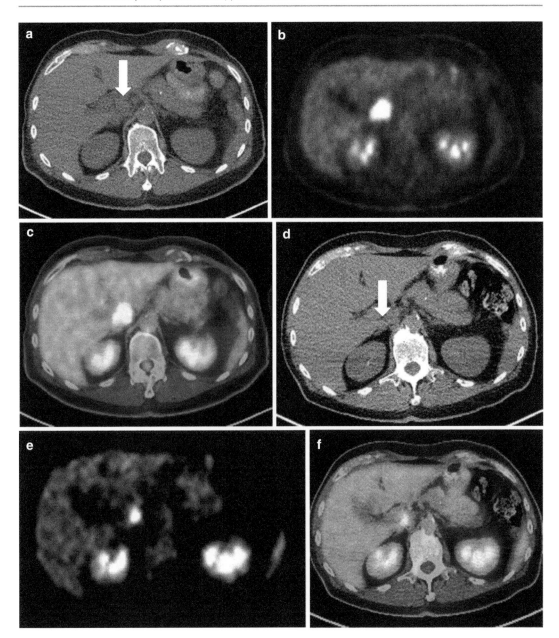

Fig. 6.7 Reduction in the size and metabolic activity of metastases following treatment of a patient with V600E BRAF containing melanoma with concurrent BRAF and MEK inhibitors. A 73-year-old male with initial PET/CT showing a 2.6 cm porta hepatis lymph (arrow) on non-contrast CT (**a**) which is FDG avid on PET image (**b**) and fused image (**c**) with a SUVmax of 22. Patient was started on dabrafenib and trametinib. Follow-up imaging 3 months later reveals the porta hepatis lymph node to have decreased in size to 1.1 cm (arrow) on non-contrast CT (**d**) as well as FDG avidity with an SUVmax of only 6.5 on PET (**e**) and fused (**f**) images

of a lesion on CT scan may not necessarily reflect growth of tumor but rather infiltration of immune cells that have potential to kill the melanoma cells. Immunotherapy can lead to responses over time despite an initial increase in size of metastatic lesions because of immune cell infiltration, a concept termed pseudo-progression. Figure 6.8 pictorially presents patterns of treatment efficacy

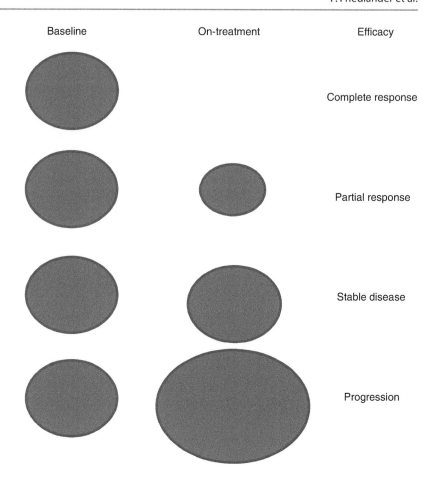

Fig. 6.8 Response patterns to treatment with cytotoxic chemotherapy or molecularly targeted therapy. Comparison of the size determined by measurement of melanoma lesions on a CT scan at baseline to the size obtained on repeat imaging several months after initiating treatment with chemotherapy or targeted therapy. The blue circles represent a metastasis. Complete shrinkage represents a complete response, partial shrinkage a partial response, no or slight change in size stable disease, and increase in size progression of disease

determined by CT imaging in the context of treatment with chemotherapy or BRAF-targeted therapy. Figure 6.9 shows variations of these patterns in the context of treatment with immunotherapy that can cause pseudo-progression.

It can be difficult to differentiate true versus pseudo-progression, but the clinical implications are extremely important as oncologists want to change treatment type if tumor is truly progressing but do not want to discontinue immunotherapy prematurely given potential for durable benefit. A strategy to help differentiate is to assess for changes in performance status and tumor-related symptoms in a patient receiving immunotherapy. If imaging performed after several months on therapy shows increases in tumor size but the patient feels well or better than pretreatment, the potential for pseudo-progression exists, and treatment can be continued with a plan for short-interval repeat in imaging 4–8 weeks later.

If further increase in tumor burden is appreciated on the short-interval repeat imaging, then true progression is considered. Pseudo-progression can occur not just extracranially but also in brain metastases followed on MR imaging [29]. Pseudo-progression has also been reported in the context of intra-lesional administration of the immune-modulatory oncolytic virus TVEC [30]. TVEC was injected into metastatic lymph nodes with 50% of the nodes demonstrating an initial increase in size from baseline that was followed by shrinkage.

To assess the efficacy of a treatment in the context of a clinical trial, the response evaluation criteria in solid tumors (RECIST) were developed [31]. RECIST classifies efficacy as complete response (CR), partial response (PR), stable disease (SD), or disease progression (PD). Determination depends on changes in tumor burden and the presence or absence of new lesions.

Fig. 6.9 Response patterns to treatment with immunotherapy. (**a**) Comparison of the size of melanoma metastasis at baseline to 12 weeks on treatment as measured by CT imaging. The blue circles represent a metastasis. Complete shrinkage represents a complete response, partial shrinkage a partial response, no or slight change in size stable disease, and increase in size either progression of disease or pseudo-progression due to immune cell infiltration. (**b**) Differentiation of true versus pseudo-progression. If tumor size is larger on week 12 imaging, CT imaging is repeated in a short interval 4–8 weeks later. A further increase in tumor size characterizes true progression, while shrinkage is consistent with the week 12 imaging showing pseudo-progression

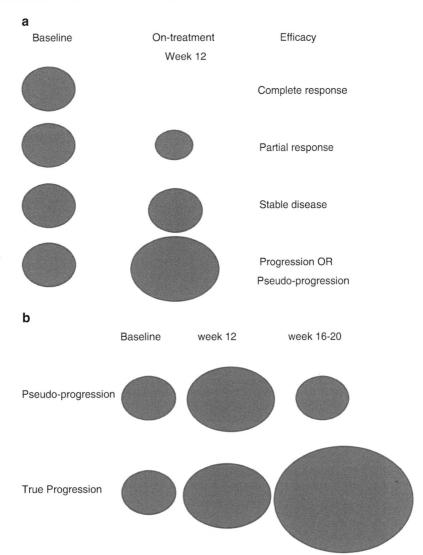

Target lesions are chosen, and changes in dimensional characteristics are summed together to determine response with an increase in the sum of unidimensional target lesion diameters of 20% or greater defining disease progression. Other lesions are termed nontarget lesions and can contribute to defining a complete response or disease progression. The development of new lesions represents disease progression. RECIST assessment was developed to assess efficacy of cytotoxic chemotherapy, but limitations can lead to underestimation of efficacy to immunotherapy. Immune checkpoint-based treatments can lead to pseudo-progression with an initial increase in the size of target and nontarget lesions leading to incorrect classification as disease progression. Similarly new lesions can develop that reflect immune cell infiltration of subclinical metastases and therefore not be due to disease progression. However RECIST would lead to treatment discontinuation on the basis of classification as progressive disease.

These limitations have led to the development of immune-modified RECIST (imRECIST) and immune-related response criteria (irRC) [32, 33]. irRC, initially published in 2009, was based on outcomes of 487 patients treated with ipilimumab as part of three multicenter phase II trials.

Induction treatment was administered every 3 weeks for a total of four treatments and then efficacy assessed at week 12 by an independent review committee review of the CT imaging. Patients with progressive disease at week 12 but remaining clinically stable were encouraged to continue treatment. Disease control was appreciated in approximately 30% of the ipilimumab-treated patients at week 12. Four different patterns of response were appreciated. The response patterns include initial tumor shrinkage and no development of new lesions, durable stable disease followed by gradual decline in metastatic tumor burden, tumor shrinkage after an initial increase in tumor size, and response in the presence of new lesions (which could represent pseudo-progression of lesions). All four of these patterns are associated with improved survival [34]. Within these four response patterns, only the patterns that did not include new lesions or increase in size of lesions would have been considered a response by traditional measurement criteria such as RECIST. The irRC was developed to increase the sensitivity of capturing responses using bidimensional measurements of target lesions multiplying the longest diameter by the longest perpendicular diameter of each lesion and summing the measurements together [34]. New measureable lesions are incorporated into tumor burden, and new nonmeasurable lesions do not constitute disease progression with progressive disease defined as at least a 25% increase in tumor burden compared with nadir in two consecutive observations at least 4 weeks apart [34].

The irRC utilizes bidimensional measurements which are cumbersome to obtain. As such a prospective analysis of 57 stage IV melanoma patients treated with ipilimumab in an expanded access phase II study was performed to compare response assessment utilizing unidimensional versus bidimensional irRC [32]. A high concordance on follow-up imaging was appreciated in percent tumor size change using unidimensional and bidimensional measurements (Spearman r: 0.953–0.965) with high concordance of best immune response between the uni- and bidimensional criteria [32]. At the same time, unidimensional measurements led to greater reproducibility.

This data suggests that irRC using unidimensional measurements are highly concordant to results seen with bidimensional measurements while being simpler to calculate with less variation.

imRECIST was developed as a modification of RECISTv1.1 to more completely capture treatment response and disease control in the context of clinical trial treatment with the PD-L1 inhibitor atezolizumab [35]. imRECIST uses unidimensional measurements with new lesions or enlarging nontarget lesions not necessarily defining progression of disease. The best overall response may occur after PD assessments. Efficacy of atezolizumab treatment in patients with advanced non-small cell lung cancer, urothelial carcinoma, renal cell carcinoma, and melanoma as part of several clinical trials was determined using imRECIST versus RECIST v1.1 criteria. Use of imRECIST led to 1–2% increase in best overall response, 8–13% increase in disease control rate, and 0.5–1.5-month improvement in median progression-free survival [35].

Response patterns and the relationship between the best overall response and the overall survival of 327 advanced melanoma patients treated with pembrolizumab on the KEYNOTE-001 study who had at least 28 weeks of imaging were compared using irRC and RECISTv1.1 criteria. Patients were treated with pembrolizumab at a dose of 2 or 10 mg/kg every 2 or 3 weeks. Seven percent of patients were found to have pseudo-progression with 5% having early and 3% delayed pseudo-progression. Fourteen percent of patients who survived at least 12 weeks (the time of initial posttreatment initiation imaging) were classified as having disease progression by RECIST v1.1 but were not progressive when irRC was used. Two-year overall survival was 37.5% in patients who had progressive disease by RECISTv1.1 but nonprogressive disease by as opposed to only 17.3% in patients classified as having disease progression by both response criteria. Therefore standard RECIST appears to underestimate benefit conferred by anti-PD-1 therapy in approximately 15% of patients [36]. Table 6.1 compares the characteristics used to define disease progression using RECIST v1.1, irRC, and imRECIST [35].

Table 6.1 Comparison of characteristics defining progression using RECIST v1.1, IrRC, and imRECIST measuring criteria

Characteristic	RECIST v1.1	irRC	imRECIST
Measurement type	Unidimensional	Bidimensional	Unidimensional
Number target lesions	Up to 5	Up to 10	Up to 5
Maximum number of target lesions per organ	2	5	2
Nontarget lesions	For CR need resolve	Increase in size does not definitely mean progression	Increase in size does not definitely mean progression
	If clear progression then PD	Add to total tumor burden measurable new lesions	Add to total tumor burden measurable new lesions
New lesions	Disease progression	Not definitely progression. If measurable add to total tumor burden	Not definitely progression. If measurable add to total tumor burden
Disease progression	20% or greater increase in sum of lesion diameters, clear progression in nontarget lesions, new lesions, 5 mm or greater increase in size from nadir	Use only measurable disease to determine Need confirm progression with repeat imaging 4 or more weeks later 0.25% or greater increase in sum of the longest diameters relative to baseline or nadir	Use only measurable disease to determine Need confirm progression with repeat imaging 4 or more weeks later 0.20% or greater increase in sum of the longest diameters relative to baseline or nadir

irRC and imRECIST allow for an increase in size of lesions or the development of new lesions without constituting disease progression to immunotherapy. This allows for increased sensitivity to detect a response given potential for immunotherapy to cause pseudo-progression

RECIST and immune-modified RECIST measurements assess efficacy of treatment in patients treated on clinical trials with the clinical trials typically requiring contrast-enhanced CT imaging to define and measure dimensions of target lesions. However in clinical practice outside of clinical trials, ^{18}F-FDG-PET/CT scans are often used by oncologists to assess melanoma treatment efficacy. A concern is that immunotherapies induce inflammatory responses that may alter ^{18}F-FDG lesional avidity. To determine if ^{18}F-FDG PET/CT can predict for prognosis in metastatic melanoma patients treated with ipilimumab, 60 consecutive ipilimumab-treated patients with metastatic melanoma obtained baseline treatment and posttreatment ^{18}F-FDG PET/CTs [37]. Response was assessed using PET response criteria in solid tumors (PERCIST5) where new concerning lesions were considered progression and by immune-modified PERCIST5 (imPERCIST5) where new lesions do not classify as progression but rather need an increase of at least 30% in the sum of lesional SUL peak (stan-

dard uptake value normalized to lean body mass). Using imPERCIST5 the 2-year survival was 66% in responders as opposed to 29% in non-responders ($p = 0.003$), and imPERCIST5 remained prognostic in multivariate analysis [37]. As such response determined on ^{18}F-FDG PET/CT may be prognostic for survival when determined but changes in the sum of SUL peak.

While response determined on PET imaging may be prognostic for ipilimumab-treated patients, response is determined after completion of four doses of ipilimumab (week 12). To determine if an earlier on-treatment ^{18}F-FDG PET/CT may predict for response, 22 patients with unresectable melanoma treated with ipilimumab had ^{18}F-FDG PET/CT performed pretreatment, after two of the planned four cycles of ipilimumab, and after completion of all four cycles [38]. The early PET/CT imaging predicted for response outcome in 18 of the 22 patients. While a limited sample size, 13 of the 15 patients who ultimately progressed were determined to progress also on the earlier on-treatment PET/CT. The other two patients were classified as stable disease on the initial on-treatment PET/CT and clearly progressed on the later on-treatment imaging [38].

Performance of ^{18}F-FDG PET/CT pretreatment, at days 21–28 post-initiation of treatment, and at 4 months on-treatment in 20 patients treated with a checkpoint inhibitor (the majority of patients were treated with ipilimumab and the remainder a PD-1 or PD-L1 inhibitor) found that early on-treatment ^{18}F-FDG PET/CT predicted eventual response with a 100% sensitivity, 93% specificity, and 95% accuracy [39]. Therefore serial ^{18}F-FDG PET/CT can play a role in staging advanced melanoma and in determining the efficacy of immune checkpoint therapy and, possibly, through early on-treatment assessment, play a prognostic role but that needs further investigation with a larger number of patients [40].

6.4   Conclusion

The overall prognosis of patients with stage IV melanoma has been improving through the development of more efficacious treatments which block inhibitory immune-regulatory checkpoints or inhibit constitutively activated BRAF. Use of immunotherapy has led to the development of novel patterns of treatment response. Enlargement of metastases on imaging may not reflect true progression but rather infiltration of immune cells. This has led to development of novel strategies which use immune criteria to measure and assess response. Roles for very early on-treatment imaging studies to assess for changes in tumor size or metabolic activity warrant further investigation to determine the potential to play a predictive role in assessing efficacy.

References

1. Siegel RL, Miller KD, Jemal A. Cancer statistics, 2018. CA Cancer J Clin. 2018;68(1):7–30.
2. Gershenwald JE, et al. Melanoma staging: Evidence-based changes in the American Joint Committee on Cancer eighth edition cancer staging manual. CA Cancer J Clin. 2017;67(6):472–92.
3. Morton DL, et al. Final trial report of sentinel-node biopsy versus nodal observation in melanoma. N Engl J Med. 2014;370(7):599–609.
4. Chapman PB, et al. Phase III multicenter randomized trial of the Dartmouth regimen versus dacarbazine in patients with metastatic melanoma. J Clin Oncol. 1999;17(9):2745–51.
5. Atkins MB, et al. High-dose recombinant interleukin-2 therapy in patients with metastatic melanoma: long-term survival update. Cancer J Sci Am. 2000;6(Suppl 1):S11–4.
6. Hodi FS, et al. Improved survival with ipilimumab in patients with metastatic melanoma. N Engl J Med. 2010;363(8):711–23.
7. Schadendorf D, et al. Pooled analysis of long-term survival data from phase II and phase III trials of ipilimumab in unresectable or metastatic melanoma. J Clin Oncol. 2015;33(17):1889–94.
8. Hamid O, et al. Five-year survival outcomes for patients with advanced melanoma treated with pembrolizumab in KEYNOTE-001. Ann Oncol. 2019;30:582–8
9. Schachter J, et al. Pembrolizumab versus ipilimumab for advanced melanoma: final overall survival results of a multicentre, randomised, open-label phase 3 study (KEYNOTE-006). Lancet. 2017;390(10,105):1853–62.
10. Topalian SL, et al. Safety, activity, and immune correlates of anti-PD-1 antibody in cancer. N Engl J Med. 2012;366(26):2443–54.
11. Larkin J, et al. Overall survival in patients with advanced melanoma who received nivolumab versus investigator's choice chemotherapy in CheckMate 037: a randomized, controlled, open-label phase III trial. J Clin Oncol. 2018;36(4):383–90.
12. Weber JS, et al. Nivolumab versus chemotherapy in patients with advanced melanoma who progressed after anti-CTLA-4 treatment (CheckMate 037): a randomised, controlled, open-label, phase 3 trial. Lancet Oncol. 2015;16(4):375–84.
13. Ascierto PA, et al. Survival outcomes in patients with previously untreated BRAF wild-type advanced melanoma treated with nivolumab therapy: three-year follow-up of a randomized phase 3 trial. JAMA Oncol. 2018; https://doi.org/10.1001/jamaoncol.2018.451.
14. Hodi FS, et al. Nivolumab plus ipilimumab or nivolumab alone versus ipilimumab alone in advanced melanoma (CheckMate 067): 4-year outcomes of a multicentre, randomised, phase 3 trial. Lancet Oncol. 2018;19(11):1480–92.
15. Hu JC, et al. A phase I study of OncoVEXGM-CSF, a second-generation oncolytic herpes simplex virus expressing granulocyte macrophage colony-stimulating factor. Clin Cancer Res. 2006; 12(22):6737–47.
16. Andtbacka RH, et al. Talimogene laherparepvec improves durable response rate in patients with advanced melanoma. J Clin Oncol. 2015;33(25):2780–8.

17. Covington MF, et al. FDG-PET/CT for monitoring response of melanoma to the novel oncolytic viral therapy talimogene laherparepvec. Clin Nucl Med. 2017;42(2):114–5.

18. Solus JF, Kraft S. Ras, Raf, and MAP kinase in melanoma. Adv Anat Pathol. 2013;20(4):217–26.

19. Davies H, et al. Mutations of the BRAF gene in human cancer. Nature. 2002;417(6892):949–54.

20. Wan PT, et al. Mechanism of activation of the RAF-ERK signaling pathway by oncogenic mutations of B-RAF. Cell. 2004;116(6):855–67.

21. Sondergaard JN, et al. Differential sensitivity of melanoma cell lines with BRAFV600E mutation to the specific Raf inhibitor PLX4032. J Transl Med. 2010;8:39.

22. Flaherty KT, et al. Inhibition of mutated, activated BRAF in metastatic melanoma. N Engl J Med. 2010;363(9):809–19.

23. Chapman PB, et al. Improved survival with vemurafenib in melanoma with BRAF V600E mutation. N Engl J Med. 2011;364(26):2507–16.

24. McArthur GA, et al. Safety and efficacy of vemurafenib in BRAF(V600E) and BRAF(V600K) mutation-positive melanoma (BRIM-3): extended follow-up of a phase 3, randomised, open-label study. Lancet Oncol. 2014;15(3):323–32.

25. Hauschild A, et al. Dabrafenib in BRAF-mutated metastatic melanoma: a multicentre, open-label, phase 3 randomised controlled trial. Lancet. 2012;380(9839):358–65.

26. Ascierto PA, et al. Cobimetinib combined with vemurafenib in advanced BRAF(V600)-mutant melanoma (coBRIM): updated efficacy results from a randomised, double-blind, phase 3 trial. Lancet Oncol. 2016;17(9):1248–60.

27. Dummer R, et al. Overall survival in patients with BRAF-mutant melanoma receiving encorafenib plus binimetinib versus vemurafenib or encorafenib (COLUMBUS): a multicentre, open-label, randomised, phase 3 trial. Lancet Oncol. 2018;19(10):1315–27.

28. Schadendorf D, et al. Three-year pooled analysis of factors associated with clinical outcomes across dabrafenib and trametinib combination therapy phase 3 randomised trials. Eur J Cancer. 2017;82:45–55.

29. Simard JL, Smith M, Chandra S. Pseudoprogression of Melanoma Brain Metastases. Curr Oncol Rep. 2018;20(11):91.

30. Zamora C, et al. Imaging manifestations of pseudoprogression in metastatic melanoma nodes injected with talimogene laherparepvec: initial experience. AJNR Am J Neuroradiol. 2017;38(6):1218–22.

31. Litiere S, et al. RECIST—learning from the past to build the future. Nat Rev Clin Oncol. 2017;14(3):187–92.

32. Nishino M, et al. Developing a common language for tumor response to immunotherapy: immune-related response criteria using unidimensional measurements. Clin Cancer Res. 2013;19(14):3936–43.

33. Seymour L, et al. iRECIST: guidelines for response criteria for use in trials testing immunotherapeutics. Lancet Oncol. 2017;18(3):e143–52.

34. Wolchok JD, et al. Guidelines for the evaluation of immune therapy activity in solid tumors: immune-related response criteria. Clin Cancer Res. 2009;15(23):7412–20.

35. Hodi FS, et al. Immune-modified response evaluation criteria in solid tumors (imRECIST): refining guidelines to assess the clinical benefit of cancer immunotherapy. J Clin Oncol. 2018;36(9):850–8.

36. Hodi FS, et al. Evaluation of immune-related response criteria and RECIST v1.1 in patients with advanced melanoma treated with pembrolizumab. J Clin Oncol. 2016;34(13):1510–7.

37. Ito K, et al. F-18 FDG PET/CT for monitoring of ipilimumab therapy in patients with metastatic melanoma. J Nucl Med. 2019;60:335–41.

38. Sachpekidis C, et al. Predictive value of early 18F-FDG PET/CT studies for treatment response evaluation to ipilimumab in metastatic melanoma: preliminary results of an ongoing study. Eur J Nucl Med Mol Imaging. 2015;42(3):386–96.

39. Cho SY, et al. Prediction of response to immune checkpoint inhibitor therapy using early-time-point (18)F-FDG PET/CT imaging in patients with advanced melanoma. J Nucl Med. 2017;58(9):1421–8.

40. Perng P, Marcus C, Subramaniam RM. (18)F-FDG PET/CT and melanoma: staging, immune modulation and mutation-targeted therapy assessment, and prognosis. AJR Am J Roentgenol. 2015;205(2):259–70.

Imaging of Dermal Trauma: Burns and Foreign Bodies

Robert L. Bard

Clinical evaluation of burn depth and wound healing remains problematic.

Burn depth may be evaluated by high-resolution sonography with copious sterile gel or a sterile standoff pad. It is also studied by technologies including near-infrared spectroscopy, thermography, nuclear radio-tracer analysis, fluorescent imaging, hyperspectral imaging, laser Doppler imaging (LDI), multiphoton microscopy (MPM), reflectance confocal microscopy (RCM), and optical coherence tomography (OCT) which are covered in-depth in later chapters. These latter systems are depth limited to 1–2 mm at the current time [1].

Burn tissue viability is quantitatively evaluated by tissue vascularity and oxygenation assessable by all the perfusion imaging modalities with the depth limitations previously described. Cicatrix generally contains abundant perilesional vascular supply allowing for better healing following reconstructive surgical procedures [2].

Burn depth is measured using standard 15–22 MHz probes and experimentally from 30 to 200 MHz and is highly reliable to find the demarcation between normal dermis and edematous tissue (Fig. 7.1). The presence of carbonized skin will appear as an echogenic region where the sonic shadowing is proportional to the extent of tissue destruction and appears similar to the iceball effect of frozen human tissue which is used as a clinical endpoint of successful thermal cryosurgery. In addition to fluid formation in the epidermis (blistering), the viability of tissue using Doppler sonography is useful (Fig. 7.2) and serially and quantitatively studied by 3D Doppler histogram analysis of the injured tissue volume (Fig. 7.3). In second-degree burns, improvement is demonstrated by decreasing edematous dermal thickness on interval imaging studies and when normalized is compared with the healthy adjacent tissue depth (Fig. 7.4). The new optical technologies with higher resolution can show microvessels (Fig. 7.5) that may be useful in skin grafts and tissue flaps to verify blood perfusion to avoid potential rejection. Infectious complications in serious burns create inflammatory new vessels that are readily imaged by sonograms as well as deeper subdermal and intramuscular abscesses which are routinely drained under ultrasound guidance procedures. Tissue oxygenation and vessel flow parameters potentially are future noninvasive spectral and hyperspectral devices for dermal health observation has not yet been fully studied in burn patients. While laser Doppler imaging (LDI) is currently used in the hospital setting, the possibility of an emergency response team carrying a portable sonogram is feasible since noncontact options are available [3]. Skin thickness is variable in anatomic sites

R. L. Bard (✉)
Director, The AngioFoundation, New York, NY, USA
e-mail: rbard@cancerscan.com;
www.angiofoundation.org

© Springer Nature Switzerland AG 2020
R. L. Bard (ed.), *Image Guided Dermatologic Treatments*,
https://doi.org/10.1007/978-3-030-29236-2_7

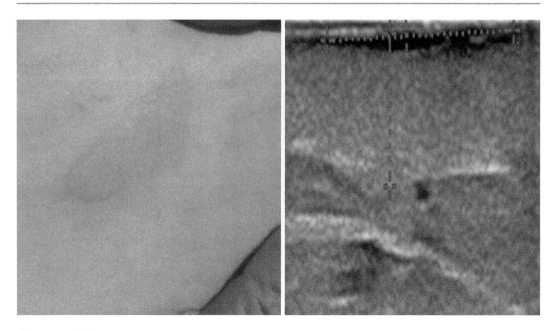

Fig. 7.1 (Left) Second-degree burn. (Right) Echo-poor burn (dotted line) extends 2.6 mm below the normal 1.3 mm dermis

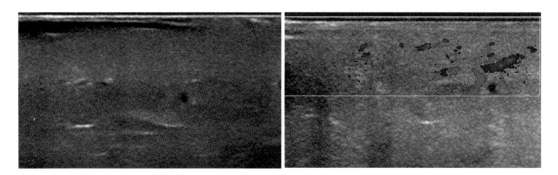

Fig. 7.2 (Left) 2D scan: fluid appears well delimited from the upper dermis. (Right) Doppler scan: reactive neovascularity extends to 4 mm depth

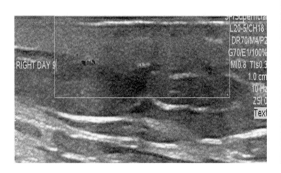

Fig. 7.3 Doppler: vessels are decreased on day 9 with edema unchanged

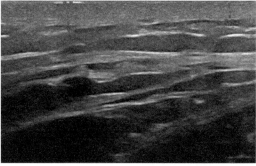

Fig. 7.4 2D scan: tissue edema reduced to 2.4 mm depth at day 15

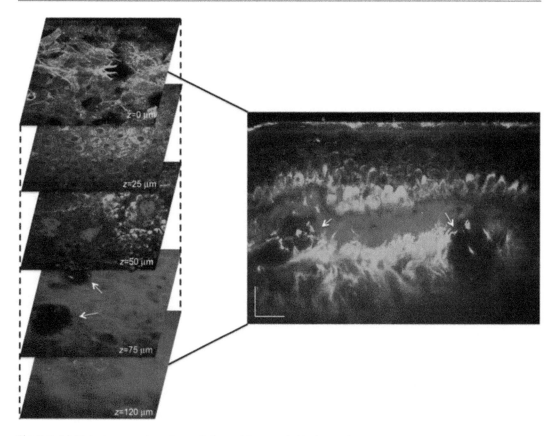

Fig. 7.5 Multiphoton scan: dermal vessels imaged in normal skin (arrows)

and does not relate directly to function. Tissue health and successful wound healing are highly correlated with the presence of stem cell-rich sweat ducts and hair follicles measurable by very high-resolution sonography and essential for re-epithelialization [4]. Recent studies have explored RCM- reflectance confocal microscopy imaging of burn [51, 52] and other wounds [53–57] to track and predict healing.

7.1 Foreign Body Imaging

Penetrating foreign bodies are common in patients visiting the emergency department; however many occur during strenuous physical activity and emotional stress that may be discounted as minor or temporary and forgotten when the pain or erythema subsides [5]. The foreign body may remain asymptomatic for long periods of time or rapidly develop a wide range of compli-

cations including pain from abscess formation, chronic discharging wound, necrotizing fasciitis, granulomas leading to bone and joint destruction including tendon infiltration with shredding and tearing, vascular events including thrombophlebitis with or without pulmonary emboli, and generalized massive soft tissue injury [6–11].

Many foreign bodies are radiographically visible if metallic or possess radiopaque content. Nonradiopaque glass and wooden fragments are often horizontally aligned with the skin surface and frequently indistinguishable on 2D sonograms from the normal fibrous septa coursing parallel to the dermis. 3D or the real-time 4D imaging shows these foreign bodies in sharp contrast to the adjacent subcutaneous or musculotendinous tissue (Figs. 7.6, 7.7, 7.8, and 7.9).

The body reacts to these intrusions by forming a protective inflammatory process which produces a circumferential sphere of echo-poor tissue that surrounds acute lesions (Figs. 7.10,

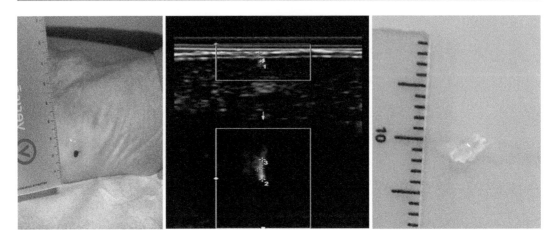

Fig. 7.6 (Left) Postop foreign body entrance site. (Middle) 2D scan: glass (top cursor #1); 3D scan glass remnant (lower cursor #2-3). (Right) Postop fragment following ultrasound-guided extraction

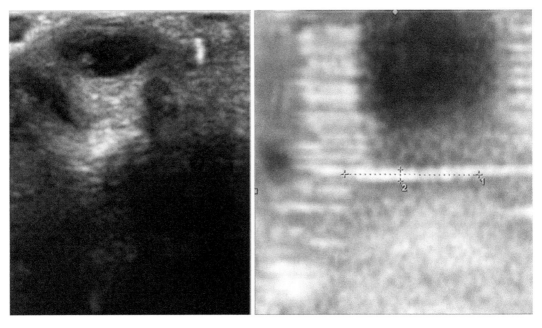

Fig. 7.7 (Left) 2D scan: zucchini plant filament (strong echoes) transverse image 0.5 mm next to dermal cyst (echo-free). (Right) 3D scan: full 6 mm length of fiber (dotted line) adjacent to cyst

7.11, and 7.12). The "halo" is echo poor sharply highlighting the more central brightly echogenic foreign body [11] representing edema, abscess, or granulation tissue (Fig. 7.13), and Doppler demonstrates peripheral neovascularity corresponding to the degree of the inflammation. In cases of less severe tissue reaction, the edema or chronic inflammatory tissue may be insufficient to spotlight the foreign body. In these instances, the object generally produces an interruption of the sound beam penetration which produces a "sonic shadow" effect that appears as a darkened vertical zone within the whiter normal tissues (Figs. 7.14, 7.15, and 7.16). An extreme example of this finding occurs when the foreign body or chronic inflammation calcifies as we see in calcific tendinitis or as in the common tropical parasitic infestations that generate subcutaneous

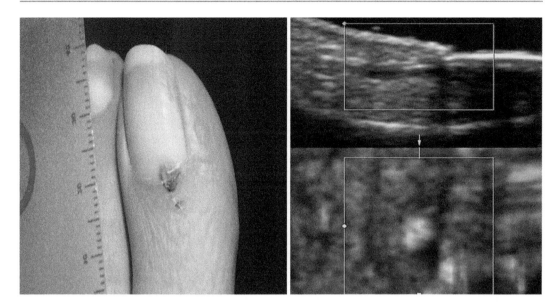

Fig. 7.8   (Left) 2-month posttrauma clinical image of pigmented lesion in suspected melanoma. (Right) 2D scan (top) sliver from fiberglass (dot, yellow): 3D gives full outline (dot, blue)

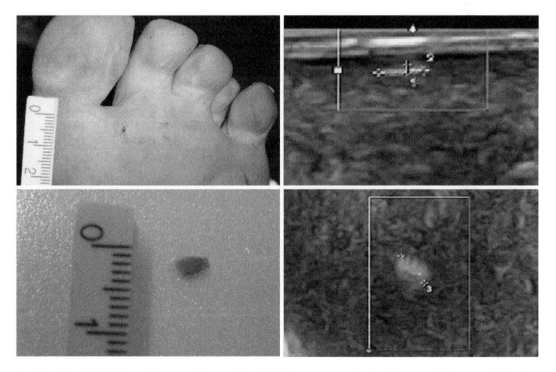

Fig. 7.9   (Top left) Clinical of pigmented lesion. (Top right) 2D shows wooden shard (cursor); 3D (bottom right) offers broader surface outline (cursor). (Bottom left) Nonradiopaque wood specimen

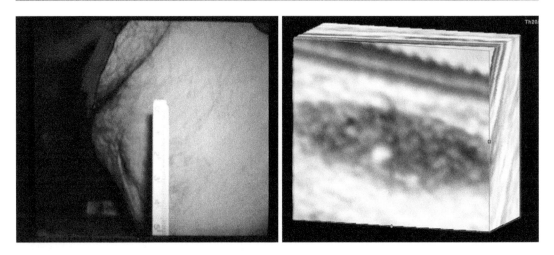

Fig. 7.10 Clinical of subdermal mass: 3D glass body reconstruction depicts wood fragment inside fibroma as oval echogenic focus central to echo-poor edema

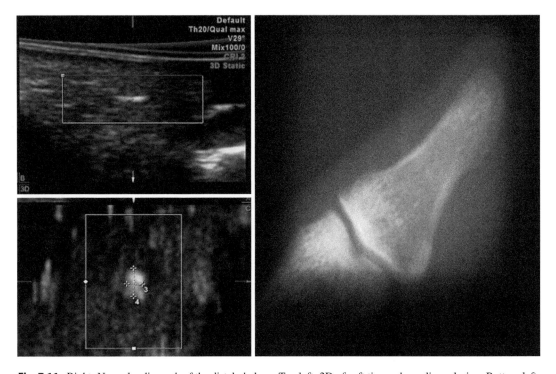

Fig. 7.11 Right: Normal radiograph of the distal phalanx. Top left: 2D of soft tissue shows linear lesion. Bottom left: 3D outlines lesion surface (cursor 3–4)

masses which are now reaching the United States due to the globalization of the planet (Fig. 7.17).

Sonography is particularly important in the extremities since weight bearing and movement affect the distribution of the foreign body in the penetrated tissues. The wood, metal, or glass may

fracture with displacement of fragments or be forced into locations unexpected by the initial portal of entry.

An intratendinous location cannot be easily imaged during surgical exploration, whereas sonography can pinpoint the site before or during

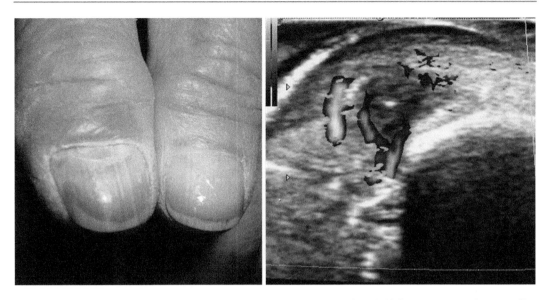

Fig. 7.12 Left: Clinical of paronychial lesion. Right: Doppler—note circumferential inflammatory vessels surrounding edema due to 0.6 mm nail fragment (arrow)—accurate depth location of 3 mm aided surgical removal

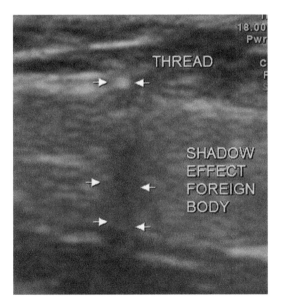

Fig. 7.13 2D of resorbable subcutaneous cosmetic thread: note sonic shadowing is only definitive finding indicated of iatrogenic foreign body

surgery with intraoperative probes. Surgical image-guided foreign body removal has been performed by the military field surgeons for over 20 years with highly reduced surgical morbidity due to the point-of-care portable sonogram units that transmit results over the Internet or satellite phone.

Foreign bodies that lie predominantly in the horizontal plane appear as linear bright echoes with or without the accompanying black shadow on standard 2D imaging. Since the 3D is multi-planar, the greatest dimension will be more easily identified in anyone of the three planes that occur simultaneously while scanning. A further refinement of 3D imaging is the 4D potential, which is real-time operator adjustment of the probe angle and position to optimize the foreign body in its most recognizable silhouette. Note how the fiberglass thread is barely distinguishable from the normal nail bed structures on 2D but appears in stark contrast to the background in the 3D version. Splinter imaging is particularly optimized by very high-frequency probes which can show the fragmented strands, perilesional fluid, and black sonic shadowing which may be missed by lower frequency probes. Significant perilesional fluid allows easier extraction of the splinter and is optimally mapped at higher frequency potentially permitting minimally invasive removal by forceps.

Similarly, intraepidermal superficial splinters may appear as pigmented lesions to the naked eye but are quickly triangulated in depth by the 2D and 3D technology. Subdermal lesions are likewise difficult to image in 2D; however the

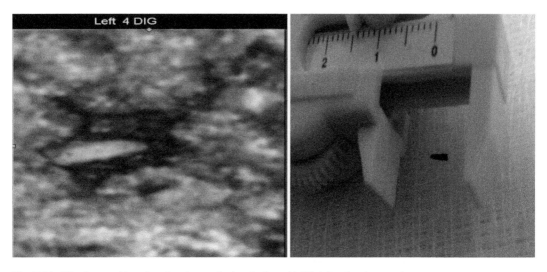

Fig. 7.14 3D of sea urchin spine showing perilesional edema highlighting 1 × 4 mm spine

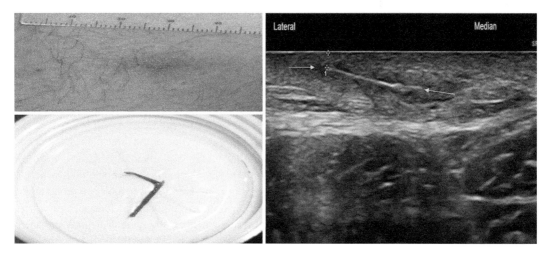

Fig. 7.15 Forearm clinical. Right: 2D demonstrates oblique descent of splinter from 1.1 mm intradermal to 2.6 mm subdermal extension. Left bottom: specimen

frequent occurrence of perilesional fluid due to local inflammatory processes creates a black background for the foreign object to be highlighted. In this case, the sea urchin spine remains uncalcified rendering radiographic imaging useless. Sonography has been used by the military of advanced countries to provide point-of-care imaging and image guidance for minimally invasive extraction techniques for over 20 years. This technology was initially developed for battlefield use by Dr. Ted Harcke for the US Army Special Forces units a quarter of a century ago [12].

Military and law enforcement trauma scars may include metallic fragments comingled with clothing fabric or the commonly used Kevlar vest. These foreign bodies may be located within the scar or several centimeters distant. The use of full-field 4 × 4 cm real-time imaging shows protective fibers at 1 cm distance from the visible scar and subdermal lesion (Fig. 7.18).

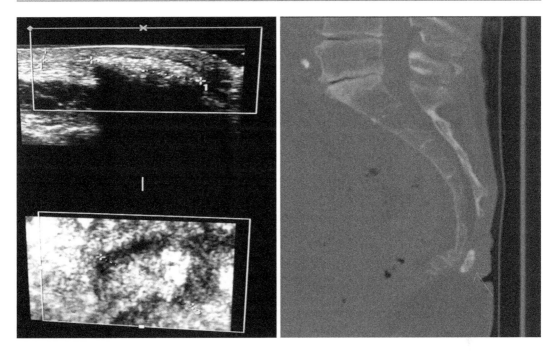

Fig. 7.16 Perianal mass palpable 2D (top) and linear echoes with sonic shadow 3D (below) outline sarcophagus of ossified *D. hominis* larva radiograph of coccyx with boney lesion (arrow)

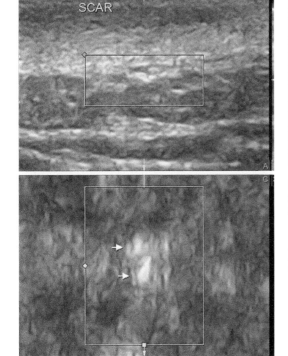

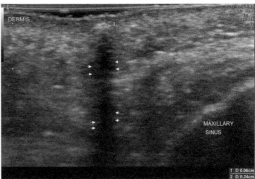

Fig. 7.18 Infraorbital intradermal foreign body: concrete fragment 0.6 mm below the epidermis length 2.6 mm—note echo-poor posttraumatic dermal echo pattern

References

1. Monstrey S, Hoeksema H, Verbelen J, et al. Assess of burn depth and healing potential. Burns. 2008;34:761–9.
2. Iftimia N, Ferguson D, Mujat M, et al. Combined reflectance confocal microscopy/optical coherence tomography imaging for skin burn assessment. Biomed Opt Express. 2013;4(5):680–95.
3. Iraniha S, Cinat M, Vanderkam V, et al. Determination of burn depth with non contact ultrasonography. J Burn Rehabil. 2000;21:333–8.

Fig. 7.17 Example of 4D scanning: shrapnel deep to scar (fragments of Kevlar vest and bullet)—the 3D boxed volume is rescanned in real time showing the two bright echoes in the subcutaneous tissues measuring 1 × 2 mm each

4. Foster F, Zhang M, Zhou Y, et al. A new ultra-sound instrument for in vivo microimaging of mice. Ultrasound Med Biol. 2000;26:63–71.
5. Tantray MD, Rather A, Gull Y, et al. Role of ultrasound in detection of radiolucent foreign bodies in extremities. Surg Trauma Limb Reconstr. 2018;13(2):81–5.
6. Fakoor M. Prolonged retention of an intramedullary wooden foreign body. Pak J Med Sci. 2006;22:78–9.
7. Freund EI, Weigl K. Foreign body granuloma: a cause of trigger thumb. J Hand Surg Br. 1984;9:210.
8. Choudhari KA, Muthu T, Tan MH. Progressive ulnar neuropathy caused by delayed migration of a foreign body. Br J Neurosurg. 2001;15:263–5.
9. Meurer WJ. Radial artery pseudoaneurysm caused by retained glass from hand laceration. Pediatr Emerg Care. 2009;25:255–7.
10. Flom LL, Ellis GL. Radiologic evaluation of foreign bodies. Emerg Med Clin North Am. 1992;10:163–76.
11. Little CM, Parker MG, Callowich MC, et al. The ultrasonic detection of soft tissue foreign bodies. Invest Radiol. 1986;21:275–7.
12. Harcke TH. Sonographic localization and management of metallic fragments. Mil Med. 2012;177:988–92.

OCT Image-Guided Treatment of Scars

8

Jill S. Waibel, Jon Holmes, Hacki Hecht, and Ashley Rudnick

8.1 Introduction

Given increased survival rates following acute traumas, the incidence of severe cutaneous scars has grown rapidly over the past decade. Injuries exceeding depths of 0.5 mm will likely result in scarring. In addition to the cosmetic defect, many scars result in hypertrophy/keloid formation, ulceration, pain, pruritus, tissue contraction, erythema, and dyspigmentation.

At the same time, scar treatment has continued to improve dramatically with the use of advanced laser technology. By creating columns of ablated tissue of precisely controlled width, depth, and density, the laser initiates a controlled wound response which results in neocollagenesis, vascular regrowth, and tissue remodeling as healthier and more normal tissue [1]. Fractional lasers have tunable pulse energies that correspond to depth. One problem with fractional lasers is that there are no clinical endpoints for

J. S. Waibel · A. Rudnick
Miami Dermatology and Laser Institute, Miami, FL, USA
e-mail: jwaibelmd@miamidermlaser.com; AshleyR@MiamiDermLaser.com

J. Holmes (✉)
Michelson Diagnostics Inc., Maidstone, Kent, UK
e-mail: jon.holmes@vivosight.com

H. Hecht
Sciton Inc., Palo Alto, CA, USA
e-mail: Hacki.Hecht@Sciton.com

the provider to monitor during treatment. Usually physicians learn through trial and error from clinical trials, colleagues, and patient successes. Dosimetry is usually estimated by the clinician with no objective data.

However, optimal outcomes are associated with matching the depth of the laser impact to the depth of the scar pathology [1–3]. The treating physician has the challenge of assessing this depth based on subjective factors such as the visual appearance of the scar and palpation. This reliance on subjective assessment can adversely impact the number of treatments required and the degree of outcome success. More objective feedback is needed to give optimal scar improvement.

VivoSight Optical Coherence Tomography (OCT) solves this problem, providing accurate, reliable measurements of scar thickness and vascular patterns in real time, enabling the laser parameters to be tuned for each treatment area and delivering enhanced results with fewer treatments. This chapter discusses the appearance of both healthy tissue and scar tissue in OCT images, and describes the methodology for interpreting the images in order to arrive at optimal laser treatment parameters. A case study is provided showing this procedure in a practical example. In summary, the VivoSight OCT scanner is a powerful new tool for the laser clinician's armamentarium for treating scar texture, enabling treatments to be better optimized to treat each patient's individual condition.

© Springer Nature Switzerland AG 2020
R. L. Bard (ed.), *Image Guided Dermatologic Treatments*,
https://doi.org/10.1007/978-3-030-29236-2_8

8.2　Scanning Protocol

As will be demonstrated in the following sections, a methodical approach for OCT assessing scar tissue is required for optimal treatment results. This approach is a complement to treatment strategies that have recently been published [1, 5].

Evaluation of the patient's scar pathology can be independent of the treatment date. It must be borne in mind that scars can be extensive lesions that have locally varying characteristics; accordingly it may be necessary to scan multiple areas and evaluate each independently.

1. **Scan procedure:** It is not necessary to use any contact gel, but ensure that the scar area is clean, dry, and free of topical medication or dressings. Touch the probe to a chosen area of the scar and when both user and patient are relaxed and ready, press the probe button to trigger a 30-s dynamic OCT scan. Capture further scans in the same manner if the scar is extended, recording the exact location of each scan each time. Also scan adjacent *normal* skin for comparison (this step may be omitted when sufficient experience has been gained).

2. **Review procedure:**
   Assess each scan in turn. First, turn off the dynamic (blood flow) overlay so that the gray structural image can be clearly seen. Initially, focus on the epidermis:
   Epidermis
   • Is the epidermis thinner or thicker than normal skin and by how much?
   • Is there a thin darker layer at the top surface (indicating thickened stratum corneum)?
   • Is the dermal-epidermal junction (DEJ) flat, slightly undulating, or highly irregular?
   Next, assess the dermis. It will be found to be useful to view both en face (top-down) and side-view displays and to adjust the depth of the en face view to reveal features of interest:
   Dermis
   • Is the DEJ "pitted"?
   • Is there a "ropy," fibrous appearance to the texture in en face view?
   • Are there patches or areas of brighter-than-normal tissue?
   Restore the dynamic (blood flow) overlay and assess the blood vessel sizes and distribution:
   • Are there areas where blood vessels are sparse or absent?
   • Measure the largest blood vessel diameters using the device on-screen measurement tool, and their depth.
   • Are the blood vessels distorted?
   Adjust the depth of the en face view to assess at what skin depth scar features "wash out" and are no longer visible. This depth is the maximum scar depth. Of course, very deep scars can exceed the OCT penetration depth, but most scars will be within measurement range.

3. **Plan treatment:** Plan the treatment, based on the characteristics of each scar area (depth, density, vascularity), employing the optimal treatment methods described in the literature [1, 5] for the type of scar and depth of scar.

4. **Repeat** the above procedure at follow-up treatment sessions. For each area of scar, carefully observe the changes in the tissue observed in OCT due to the treatment and correlate with the treatments. Keep a log showing which treatments worked best and which did not, for future reference and to guide further treatments.

8.3　Interpretation of OCT Images of Healthy Skin

Before reviewing OCT images of scar tissue, it is important to understand how healthy skin appears in OCT to be able to recognize the commonest physiological structures, including the epidermis, dermis, adnexal structures, and vessels.

VivoSight OCT produces a high-resolution vertical cross section of the skin. Because OCT uses a laser beam instead of sound, the images are of much higher resolution than is available from ultrasound (about 10× higher), but the size of the imaged region and the depth of penetration are smaller. VivoSight OCT provides images 6 mm wide with a depth penetration of ~1 mm, in real time. No contact gel is required, the user simply places the probe in contact with the skin to see the image on the device monitor. In addition, the device can be set to rapidly (30 s) scan a 6 mm × 6 mm area of skin to produce a 3-D block of data that can be viewed vertically or from above (termed "en face").

Figures 8.1a, 8.1b, and 8.1c shows annotated OCT sample images of healthy, normal skin.

8.4　Interpretation of OCT Images of Scars

Scar tissue appears differently from healthy tissue in OCT. Depending on the type of scar, severity, age, and original cause of the scar, these differences may be very obvious in the OCT image, or more subtle.

Key objectives in viewing the OCT images of scars are:

- To help assess the **nature** of the subsurface changes to the skin, to guide **type** of treatment(s)
- To measure the **depth** of the scar, to guide **depth** of laser treatment for optimal treatment

8.4.1   Hypertrophic Scars in OCT

Hypertrophic scars are those in which collagen production has been overstimulated. Collagen is overproduced producing denser, less flexible skin tissue which may protrude above surrounding normal skin. With OCT, the following features are typically observed in hypertrophic scars (Figs. 8.2a, 8.2b, 8.2c, and 8.2d).

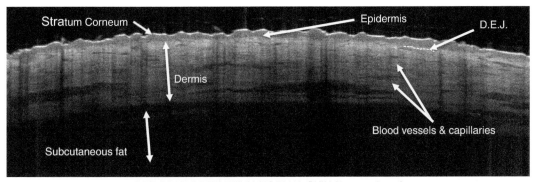

OCT SCAN OF HEALTHY, NORMAL SKIN (6 mm x 2 mm)

Fig. 8.1a OCT image size 6 mm wide × 2 mm deep. Skin of upper arm, healthy 50-year-old male

- *Stratum corneum:* The stratum corneum is extremely thin, typically 10–15 μm, and is visible in OCT as a very bright, thin layer on the very top surface.
- *Epidermis:* Below the stratum corneum, the epidermis is generally easily distinguished as a surface layer, *continuous* band with distinct darker contrast to the papillary dermis (at the dermal-epidermal junction, "DEJ"). Typically, the epidermis has a thickness of about 80–100 μm, but this varies by anatomical location.

- *Dermis:* Brighter dermis contrasting with darker epidermis. Thickness varies from 300 μm in eyelid to 1 mm+ over much of the body. In this example (upper arm) dermis is ~750 μm thick. Papillary dermis extends 200–300 μm below epidermis and is sometimes visible (as in this example) as a slightly brighter region above the reticular dermis. Blood vessels are visible as thin dark streaks; these are slightly larger in the reticular dermis than in the papillary dermis.
- *Subcutaneous layer:* Subcutaneous fat may sometimes be visible as large dark bands.

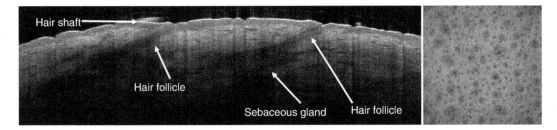

Fig. 8.1b *Adnexal Structures (left)*: Hair follicles and glands are recognized through distinct local changes in contrast that follows the physical shape of the structure. Hair follicles appear as dark streaks that are always diagonally oriented through the dermis; the hair itself can be seen as brighter streak that exits through the epidermis. The hair bulb is usually located too deep to image. Often

the hair follicle is associated with a dark oval structure deeper in the dermis, which is the sebaceous gland. (*Right*): Top view ("en face") of the OCT scan at the level of the papillary dermis layer (150 μm depth) shows hair follicles as dark dots surrounded by a medium gray halo, whereas pores appear as smaller dark dots without haloes. Image size 6 mm × 6 mm

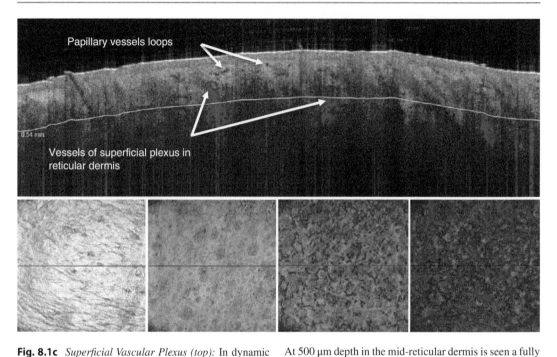

Fig. 8.1c *Superficial Vascular Plexus (top):* In dynamic OCT mode, blood cells moving through blood vessels and capillaries are detected and displayed as a red overlay. Small red dots and blobs correspond to tiny vertical blood loops in the papillary dermis. Deeper down in the reticular dermis at 300–500 μm, strong red areas indicate the presence of horizontal vessels of the superficial dermal plexus (vertical streaks are shadowing artifacts and can be ignored)

(Bottom row): Viewed in en face mode, the vessel morphology is clearly revealed. *(Left to right)*: en face scans at skin surface, at depth 150 μm (in papillary dermis), at depth 300 μm (top of reticular dermis), and at depth 500 μm (mid-reticular dermis). In the papillary dermis, fine red dots surrounding the hair follicles and pores indicate the presence of papillary loops. At the top of the reticular dermis, vessel-like fragments indicate the intersection of the imaging plane with the superficial plexus.

At 500 μm depth in the mid-reticular dermis is seen a fully developed interconnected network of vessels.

Summary of appearance of tissue constituents in OCT images:

- *Collagen* is strongly scattering to OCT and so appears bright in the image. The denser the collagen the brighter the appearance in the OCT image. Young, healthy skin appears brighter than old, photodamaged skin with less collagen. However, scar tissue may appear brighter still.
- *Keratin* appears extremely bright (often white).
- *Water* (e.g., in blisters or cysts) and edema appear as black or very dark in OCT.
- *Blood* appears as mid-gray to dark gray.
- ***Fat*** appears as mid- to dark gray, sometimes with thin bright walls to the globules
- ***Muscle*** is mid-gray—rarely seen due to depth

Fig. 8.2a Clinical image of trauma scar on thigh incurred in a boating accident

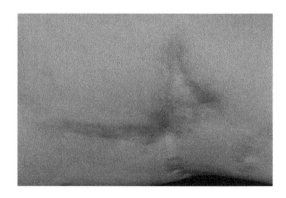

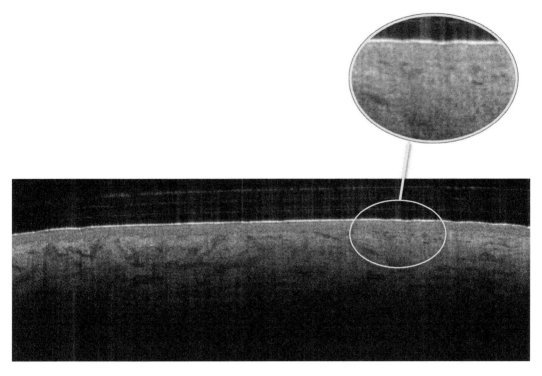

Fig. 8.2b Side-view OCT image. In the magnified inset can be seen a thin dark surface layer (stratum corneum) and flat DEJ

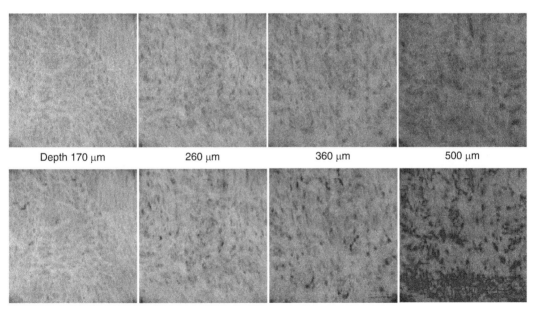

Fig. 8.2c En face images. The dermis en face image has a ropy texture which "washes out" at 500 μm. Sparse dilated, distorted blood vessels are seen to a depth of at least 500 μm. The larger vessels have diameter of approximately 150 μm

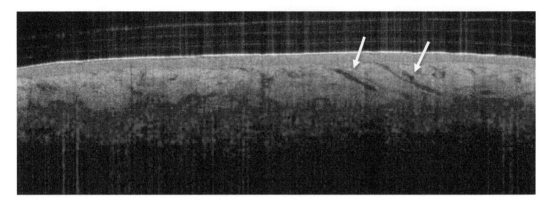

Fig. 8.2d In the dynamic overlay view, diagonal vessels reaching up to the DEJ are clearly seen (arrowed) which, coupled with thickened, flat epidermis, are typical of hypertrophic scars
OCT indicates initial treatment of this scar with PDL, or IPL with red filter, with pulse duration of 10 ms and relatively high fluence to reach the deep dermis. Nd:YAG could also be utilized if the redness does not fully respond, as this wavelength reaches deeper. Following treatment of the vessels, fractional ablative laser is used to treat the dermis. The ropy texture is visible to 300–400 μm in en face OCT view (see above) indicating a treatment depth in that range with density of 5%. Multiple treatments will be required.

8.4.1.1 Epidermis

- The epidermis is thickened compared to normal skin.
- The top surface is flatter and smoother compared to normal skin.
- The stratum corneum is often thickened, visible as a thin dark layer at the top of the epidermis.
- The DEJ is flat, whereas in normal skin the DEJ is gently undulating.

8.4.1.2 Dermis

- Shallow, dilated blood vessels are observed diagonally approaching and meeting the DEJ. This is highly characteristic of hypertrophic scars; in healthy skin, vessels in the superficial plexus are horizontal and do not approach the DEJ.
- Deeper in the dermis, isolated, large diameter, distorted vessels are observed.
- The upper dermis may exhibit a ropy, fibrous appearance.
- Areas of high collagen content appear as brighter gray patches which are vessel poor. Often, these brighter areas are surrounded by irregular dilated vessels.

8.4.2 Atrophic Scars in OCT

Atrophic scars exhibit underproduction of collagen, resulting in depressed skin surface with reduced skin flexibility. With OCT, the following features are typically observed in atrophic scars (Figs. 8.3a, 8.3b, and 8.3c).

8.4.2.1 Epidermis

- The epidermis is somewhat thinner than normal tissue.
- The DEJ may be flat.

8.4.2.2 Dermis

- There will be irregular, patchy appearance to the dermis in en face view with dynamic overlay off. These bright patches may extend deep into the dermis (the depth should be measured).
- Brighter patches will be vessel poor, but likely to be surrounded by high-density vessels directed towards the patches; sometimes these are distorted and may appear in layers.

Fig. 8.3a Acne scars on chest

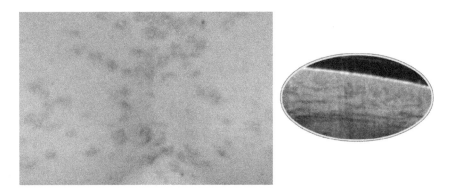

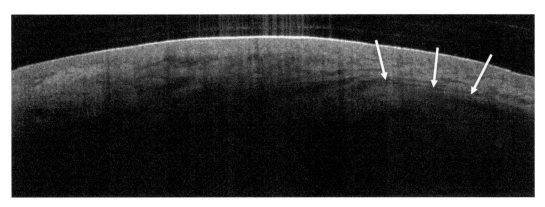

Fig. 8.3b Side view with inset showing irregular DEJ. At bottom right is a "dome" of brighter, homogeneous material which corresponds to a collagen "nodule" (arrows)

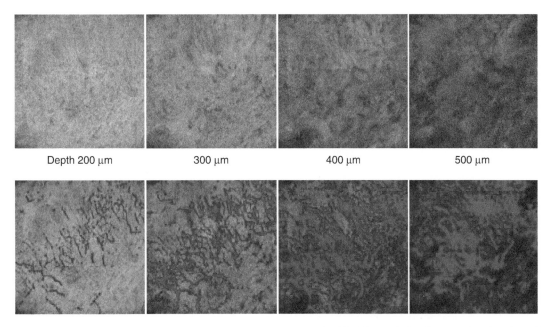

Depth 200 μm   300 μm   400 μm   500 μm

Fig. 8.3c En face views with and without dynamic overlay showing vessels

With dynamic overlay off, irregular swirls and patches are visible to at least 500 μm depth. The scar is strongly vascular with vessels as shallow as 200 μm deep in diameter range of 100–150 μm indicating a pulse duration of 3–5 ms. These vessels appear in a layer above the collagen "nodule." After treating the vessels, the deep dermis should be treated with fractional laser to a depth of at least 500 μm

8.5 Treatment Selection Based on OCT

In this chapter, we focus on the use of OCT imaging to select laser parameters, but it should be borne in mind that other treatments may be appropriate in combination or as an alternative, and the images may be valuable for these also. The objective for the treatment of hypertrophic scars is to treat to depth and with optimal laser parameters so that the scar is neither under- nor overtreated. Overtreatment may lead to more scarring or complications such as hypopigmentation.

The scar is treated in three stages: (i) epidermis, (ii) vascular, and (iii) dermis.

8.5.1 Treating the Epidermis

It is beneficial to first treat the epidermis as this is clinically most visible. Typically the abnormal epidermis will have a different micro-texture surface topography from the surrounding normal skin and this is one reason the scar is so visible. This micro-texture reflects the subsurface flexibility of the dermis which is usually lower than surrounding skin. Treating the epidermis may help trigger remodeling processes which when proceeding in parallel with laser remodeling of the dermis may tend towards that of more normal skin. It is also desirable to restore the epidermis to normal thickness and regularity. The treatment aggressiveness should accordingly be tuned to the thickness of the epidermis, as measured by OCT.

8.5.2 Treating the Vascular Component

Scars often appear pink due to vascular component and this area is the initial treatment site. OCT is first used to measure the depth of the vessels and their diameter. It may be useful to com-

Table 8.1 Laser pulse duration selection based on the theory of selective thermolysis

Diameter/µm	<50	50–100	101–160	161–250	>250
Pulse duration/ms	1	3–5	10–15	15–20	30–40

pare the dynamic OCT images of scar tissue with those of nearby tissue, in order to identify exactly *why* the scar appears pink: it may be due to large-diameter vessels deeper in the dermis, or a proliferation of small vessels at shallow depths. Often scars have regions of vessel-poor, dense collagen surrounded or enveloped by mesh layer of dilated vessels. This vascular region is the next area to be targeted. To treat these vessels, the principles of selective photothermolysis by Anderson and Parrish should be followed to select the pulse diameter, using pulse dye laser (PDL) or intense pulsed light (IPL) for treating <400 µm depths and Nd:YAG for greater depths. The fluence used then depends on the target depth and the wavelength, with higher fluences required for deeper vessels and lower for shallow vessels. Target the largest vessels with longer pulse durations and then progress to smaller vessels as necessary in later treatment sessions (Table 8.1).

8.5.3 Treating Dermal Collagen

Treating the dermal collagen is also required to excite remodeling processes. The principal goal is to treat to the required depth, and OCT is used to assess this by observing, in the en face view, the depth at which irregular bright patches (which correspond to dense ordered collagen from scar tissue) "wash out." Once again, it may be helpful to compare with scans of nearby normal skin. Either ablative fractional laser (AFL) or non-ablative fractional laser (NAFL) modalities may be used; please refer to consensus guidelines [ref] for details. In general, low fractional densities are used for best results.

8.6   Discussion

These and many other cases scanned with OCT and then successfully treated at Miami Dermatology and Laser Institute demonstrate the power of the technique. We repeatedly observed that subsurface scar tissue is highly variable in terms of collagen structure/density, and vascular structure. Often this variation cannot be judged by eye, but is easily seen with OCT.

Scanning with OCT can be quickly performed (30 s per scan location) and can be delegated under supervision to a trained operative, for optimal practice workflow. Patient informed consent should always be obtained beforehand. The interpretation of scans should however be done by the lead physician who is treating the patient and should be done with full knowledge of the patient's medical history.

Key objectives in reviewing the OCT scans are to assess the type of scar tissue and its depth. Then treatment is designed around these two parameters, using current best practice [1–5].

The complexity of scars requires a systematic, methodical approach. Careful mapping of the scar, recording observations, enables an understanding of the whole scar leading to carefully planned treatments for optimal results.

Repeating the OCT scans at follow-up treatment sessions enables objective assessment of the impact of the preceding treatment. This helps guide further treatments, building on the knowledge gained each time.

8.7   Conclusion

The VivoSight OCT scanner is a powerful new tool for the laser clinician's armamentarium for treating scar texture, enabling treatments to be better optimized to treat each patient's individual condition. The key benefit of the OCT image guidance is the provision of real-time assessment of scar tissue character and accurate measurements of burn and trauma damage thickness and underlying vascular patterns enabling controlled treatment tuned to maximize enhanced therapy on each area of scar tissue.

References

1. Anderson R, Donelan M, Hivnor C, Greeson E, Ross V, Shumaker P, Uebelhoer N, Waibel J. Laser treatment of traumatic scars with an emphasis on ablative fractional laser resurfacing. JAMA Dermatol. 2014;150(2):187–93.
2. Waibel JS, Rudnick AC, Wulkan AJ, Holmes JD. The diagnostic role of optical coherence tomography (OCT) in measuring the depth of burn and traumatic scars for more accurate laser dosimetry: pilot study. J Drugs Dermatol. 2016;15(11): 1375–80.
3. Bowen R. A novel approach to ablative fractional treatment of mature thermal burn scars. J Drugs Dermatol. 2009;9:389–92.
4. Cohen JL. Minimizing skin cancer surgical scars using ablative fractional Er:YAG laser treatment. J Drugs Dermatol. 2013;12:1171–3.
5. Eilers R, Ross V, Cohen J, Ortiz A. A combination approach to surgical scars. Dermatol Surg. 2016;42:S150–6.

Advantages of Sonography in Fillers and Complications

9

Fernanda A. Cavallieri

9.1 Introduction

The use of cosmetic fillers has grown in recent times primarily because of the possibility of achieving aesthetic results previously only achieved with surgery.

According to data from the American Society of Plastic Surgeons (ASPS), more than 2.6 million soft tissue filler procedures were performed in 2016, making them the second most popular minimally invasive procedure performed in the USA, right after botulin toxin injections.

The identification of previous fillers in patients, as well as the evaluation and proper conduct of possible complications, is a daily challenge for dermatologists and plastic surgeons.

Therefore, ultrasonography has been shown to be an important tool in the study of cosmetic fillers, allowing the identification of fillers, as well as assisting in the evaluation and follow-up of adverse effects.

There are conflicting concepts regarding the duration and biodegradation time of cosmetic fillers. But in general, a filler can be categorized in terms of biodegradable (moderate and long duration) versus its nonbiodegradable nature. Biodegradable fillers include hyaluronic acid, poly-L-lactic acid, and calcium hydroxylapatite, while nonbiodegradable fillers include polymethyl methacrylate, polyacrylamide hydrogel, and silicone oil.

Although not being categorized as fillers, this chapter will also cover the sonographic aspects of lifting threads, which may also be biodegradable or nonbiodegradable.

9.2 Sonographic Features of Fillers

9.2.1 Hyaluronic Acid (HA)

Hyaluronic acid-based gel fillers, the most widely used biodegradable fillers in both the USA and Europe, are constituted of linear polymeric dimers of N-acetylglucosamine and glucuronic acid.

On sonography HA deposits appear as round, oval, or elongated anechoic structures, configuring a "pseudocystic" appearance (Fig. 9.1). The deposits are usually located in the subcutaneous tissue, varying only its depth. When mixed with lidocaine, it may present inner echoes within the pseudocystic structures. High-density HA presents as small- to medium-sized anechoic pseudocystic structures and is usually located in the deep hypodermis or close to the periosteum, while low-density HA presents as small-sized pseudocystic structures located superficially in the hypodermis. High-density HA deposits seem

F. A. Cavallieri (✉)
Clinica Cavallieri, Rio de Janeiro, Brazil

© Springer Nature Switzerland AG 2020
R. L. Bard (ed.), *Image Guided Dermatologic Treatments*,
https://doi.org/10.1007/978-3-030-29236-2_9

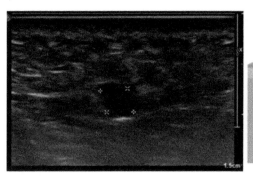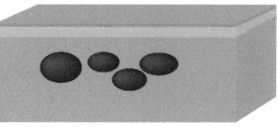

Fig. 9.1 Left: Ultrasonographic image of HA (hyaluronic acid) permeation deposit at the subcutaneous cellular tissue in the malar region (between × and +). Right: Illustrative figure of the ultrasonographic appearance of HA deposits restricted to the subcutaneous cellular tissue

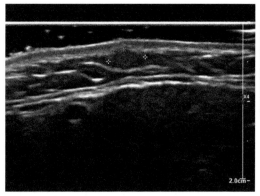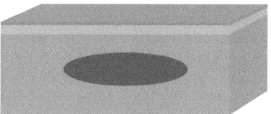

Fig. 9.2 Left: Ultrasonographic image of polylactic acid nodule at the subcutaneous cellular tissue in the malar region (between + and +). Right: illustrative figure of the ultrasonographic appearance of polylactic acid nodule restricted to the subcutaneous cellular tissue

to last longer than low-density ones and may present effects that apparently last more than 2 years [1].

vascularization on color Doppler (Fig. 9.2). The PLLA nodule is generally located in the dermis or superficial layers of the hypodermis.

9.2.2 Poly-ʟ-Lactic Acid (PLLA)

Injectable PLLA is a biocompatible, biodegradable, biostimulatory, synthetic filler that may be injected into the reticular dermis or subcutaneous fat. It stimulates neocollagenesis through fibroblast activation [2].

Usually, PLLA shows no specific aspect on ultrasound; however, in cases where it appears as palpable small nodules on injection sites, sonography shows round or oval well-defined isoechoic nodules, presenting internal and/or peripheral

9.2.3 Calcium Hydroxylapatite (CaHA)

Calcium hydroxylapatite is also a biostimulatory filler that contains microspheres which may stimulate the endogenous production of collagen. The CaHA microspheres are suspended in the carrier gel composed of sodium carboxymethylcellulose, water, and glycerin mix allowing the particles to be easily delivered upon injection [3].

On ultrasound, CaHA appears as hyperechoic deposits that may present as a continuous and sinu-

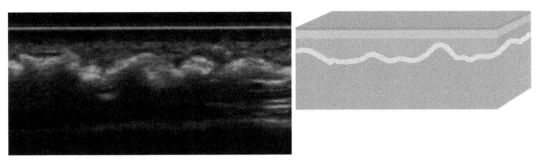

Fig. 9.3 Left: Ultrasonographic image of calcium hydroxylapatite filler at the subcutaneous cellular tissue. Right: Illustrative figure of the ultrasonographic appear- ance of calcium hydroxylapatite restricted to the subcuta- neous cellular tissue

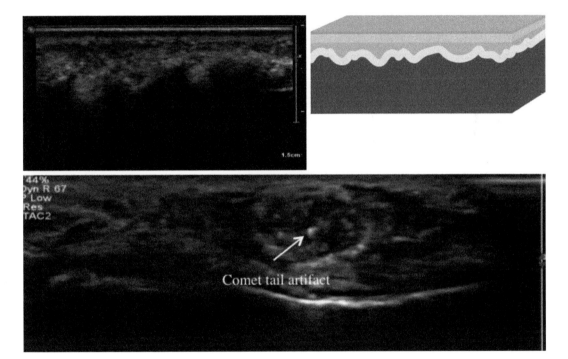

Fig. 9.4 Top left: Ultrasonographic image of polymethyl methacrylate filler at the subcutaneous cellular tissue forming a contiguous anfractuous layer. Top right: Illustrative figure of the ultrasonographic appearance of polymethyl methacrylate filler. Bottom: Hyperechoic dots producing a mini comet-tail artifact (small posterior reverberance) (arrow)

ous layer, with variable degrees of posterior acous- tic shadowing (Fig. 9.3). CaHA is usually injected in superficial layers of subcutaneous tissue.

9.2.4 Polymethyl Methacrylate (PMMA)

PMMA consists of polymethyl methacrylate microspheres suspended in a water-based gel with collagen, hyaluronic acid, or other colloidal vehicles. On ultrasound, PMMA appears as a hyperechoic continuous anfractuous layer, or focal deposits, constituted by multiple bright hyperechoic dots producing a mini comet tail- shaped artifact (posterior reverberance) (Fig. 9.4). PMMA usually produces less posterior acoustic shadowing artifacts than CaHA; nevertheless, over time (more than 6 months after injection), some of the larger filler deposits may acquire more intense posterior acoustic shadowing artifacts.

9.2.5 Polyacrylamide Hydrogel (PAAG)

Polyacrylamide filler is a nonabsorbable hydrogel consisting of 97.5% water and 2.5% cross-linked polyacrylamide hydrogel (PAAG). The gel is manufactured through polymerization of the acrylamide monomers and N,N'-methylenebisacrylamide. On ultrasound, PAAG deposits present as anechoic pseudocystic structures that may or not present debris in suspension inside, associated with increased echogenicity of the subcutaneous tissue (Fig. 9.5). In general, PAAG deposits are larger than hyaluronic acid deposits, and the latter decrease their size over time, while PAAG deposits remain with the stable dimensions.

9.2.6 Silicone Oil

In cosmetic procedures, silicone can be found in two forms: pure silicone and silicone oil. On ultrasound, pure silicone presents an anechoic oval aspect that does not change in shape or size over time. On the other hand, silicone oil appears as a hyperechoic continuous deposit, forming a layer injected right under the dermis, causing a specific posterior acoustic reverberation artifact, with a blurry white pattern, named "snowstorm" pattern (Fig. 9.6).

9.2.7 Complications

An ideal filler is cosmetically effective, neither allergenic nor immunogenic; injectable with reproducible techniques and results, with high potential for use and low for abuse; noncarcinogenic; nonteratogenic; nonmigratory; cost effective; physiologic; and permanent [4].

Unfortunately, this ideal substance does not exist. And although there are far more successful reports, as the number of procedure reports rises, the number of complications will likely also increase.

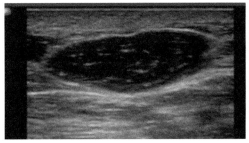 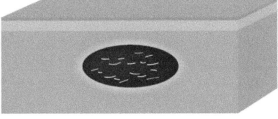

Fig. 9.5 Left: Ultrasonographic image of polyacrylamide gel filler deposit at the subcutaneous cellular tissue. Right: Illustrative figure of the ultrasonographic appearance of polyacrylamide gel filler

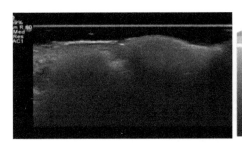 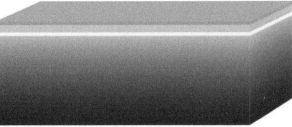

Fig. 9.6 Left: Ultrasonographic image of silicone oil filler forming a hyperechoic continuous layer, with a broad posterior reverberation artifact called "snowstorm" pattern. Right: Illustrative figure of the ultrasonographic appearance of silicone oil filler

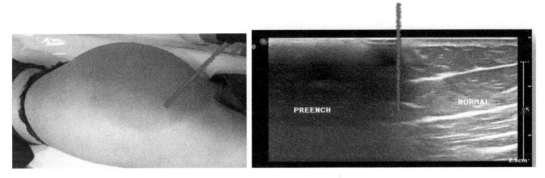

Fig. 9.7 Left: Morphea-like dermatopathy. Right: Red line marks the exact limit between presence of filler (silicone oil) and normal subcutaneous tissue, in concordance with clinical picture

The FDA (Food and Drug Administration) officially classifies these cosmetic fillers as devices, not medications. Therefore, the same precautions taken with implantable devices should be taken with fillers [5].

Complications are more frequent in patients who already have a previous filler (commonly a nondegradable one) and are injected by a second type of filler, degradable or nondegradable, in the same anatomic region. HA fillers have the very beneficial quality of responding to hyaluronidase, which allows the physician to remove the material. Nevertheless, unwanted side effects with irreversible fillers are much more difficult to manage, given that total extraction of the filler product may not be possible.

Generally, complications are divided by the onset of adverse event: early events (occurring up to several days post injection) and delayed events (occurring from weeks to years post injection).

This chapter addresses the complications in which ultrasonography plays an important role in diagnosis and management, including dermatopathies, filler migration, hypersensitivity reactions, inflammatory nodules (abscess, granulomas, and panniculitis), noninflammatory nodules ("clumps"), and vascular complications.

9.2.8 Dermatopathies

The dermatopathies associated with dermal fillers described in the literature are morphea-like (cutaneous scleroderma) and angioedema-like dermatopathies. They are associated with previous injection of nondegradable fillers, specially silicone oil, and may appear after months or years of injection. On ultrasound, morphea-like dermatopathy shows the presence of the filler respecting exactly the limits of the cutaneous lesion, prompting the clinical conclusion that its presence is the cause of the lesion (Fig. 9.7).

9.2.9 Filler Migration

Cosmetic material may migrate into areas adjacent to the injection sites, causing swollen areas or palpable masses in the vicinity of injected sites. Furthermore, it is possible to find nondegradable material in local lymph nodes near injected areas, commonly silicone oil which may traverse significant tissue distances.

9.2.10 Hypersensitivity Reactions

Those reactions may appear right after injection or be delayed by weeks to months after introduction generally appearing as erythematous rashes and early or late swellings. Sonography plays an important role in the assessment of late-stage eruptions, often intermittent and persistent, as long as the filler is present in the tissue. On ultrasound, the common characteristic in all cases of late swellings is the presence of

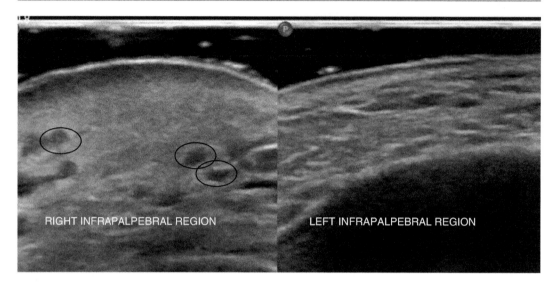

RIGHT INFRAPALPEBRAL REGION   LEFT INFRAPALPEBRAL REGION

Fig. 9.8 Hypersensitivity reaction: late swelling of right infrapalpebral region after injection of hyaluronic acid (dark circles). Sonographic images of the area showed increased echogenicity and thickening of the subcutaneous cellular tissue

the filler, associated with increased echogenicity and thickening of the surrounding subcutaneous cellular tissues (Fig. 9.8). No solid nodules or fluid collections are identified; therefore, the hypotheses of other adverse reactions characterized by the presence of nodules, abscesses, or collections are excluded [6].

9.2.11 Inflammatory Nodules

Inflammatory nodules are classified as early or delayed adverse reactions characterized by the presence of clinically palpable nodules in association with phlogistic findings. Inflammatory nodules include abscesses, chronic foreign body reactions (granulomas), and panniculitis. Ultrasound examination plays an important role in these cases, given that each nodule presents specific sonographic features. Abscess may be an early or late complication and on ultrasound is characterized as a fluid collection, with or without debris in suspension, uni- or multiloculated. On color Doppler abscesses present increased neovascularization in the surrounding tissue (Figs. 9.9 and 9.10). Chronic foreign body reactions are delayed complications, defined as granulomas on histopathology.

On ultrasound, these nodules are characterized by poorly defined, iso- or hypoechoic nodules or masses, with the presence of vascularization within and around the lesion, suggesting the presence of a chronically inflamed tissue (Fig. 9.11).

On ultrasound, panniculitis presents as a focal area of thickening of the subcutaneous cellular tissue, with increased echogenicity and laminar anechoic bands of fluid in the periphery of fatty lobules. Color Doppler ultrasound shows increased vascularization of the area and its vicinity (Fig. 9.12) [7].

9.2.12 Noninflammatory Nodules

Noninflammatory nodules are defined as product accumulations, without phlogistic signs. Usually referred as "clumps" in the literature, those accumulations are an early consequence of overfilling (injection of an excessive amount of material or a too superficial injection of filler) or possibly a delayed complication. On ultrasound, these nodules show the presence of the specific filler material, configuring a palpable nodule, without increase in the vascularization on color Doppler ultrasound.

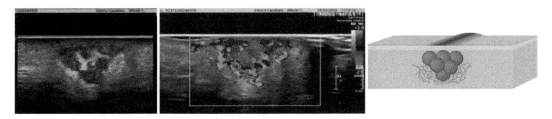

Fig. 9.9 Abscess. Left: Ultrasonographic image showing a multiloculated fluid collection with debris in suspension after injection with hyaluronic acid. Middle: color Doppler showing increase in vascularization in the surrounding tissue. Right: Illustrative figure of the ultrasonographic appearance of abscess

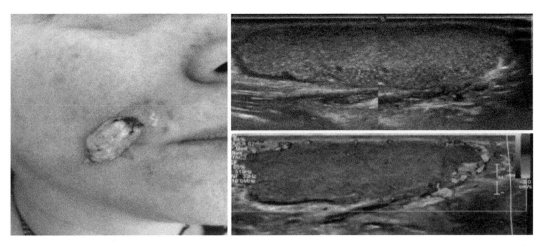

Fig. 9.10 Abscess. Left: Picture of draining abscess. Patient had hyaluronic acid injections at the nasolabial folds 3 weeks prior to picture. Right: Ultrasonographic images of fluid collection with debris in suspension with surrounding vascularization on color Doppler

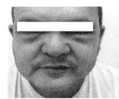 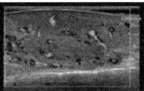 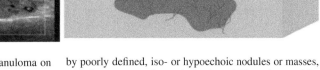

Fig. 9.11 Chronic foreign body reaction (granuloma on histopathology). Left: Picture of a patient presenting hard and erythematous nodules in infrapalpebral regions. Middle: On ultrasound, those nodules are characterized by poorly defined, iso- or hypoechoic nodules or masses, with the presence of vascularization within and around the lesion. Right: Illustrative figure of the ultrasonographic appearance of granuloma

9.2.13 Vascular Complications

Vascular complications are rare and include injection site necrosis secondary to intravascular injection of filler or external compression of blood supply. Currently, those complications have been reported in literature after HA injections. The most affected arteries are the angular artery of the nasolabial fold and the supratrochlear artery in the glabellar region [5].

Color Doppler ultrasound is an important tool in the early detection of vascular obstruction,

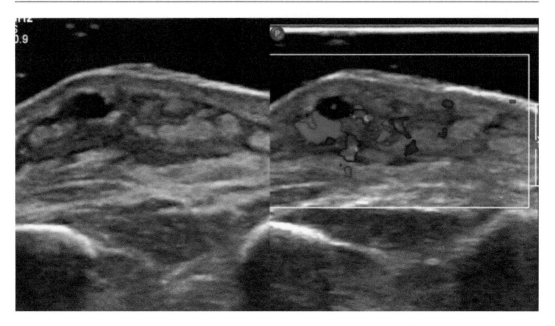

Fig. 9.12 Panniculitis. Ultrasonographic image presenting area of thickening of the subcutaneous cellular tissue, with increased echogenicity and laminar anechoic bands of fluid in the periphery of fatty lobules. Color Doppler ultrasound shows increased vascularization of the area and its vicinity

demonstrating the absence of intraluminal flow, thus confirming the diagnosis. In addition, if the filler injected was HA, ultrasound can guide intravascular hyaluronidase injection, in the exact site of thrombosis, improving the patient's prognosis [8].

9.2.14 Thread-Lifting Technique

Threads are marketed as an alternative to more invasive procedures such as a facelift, due to the long recovery time or cost-associated surgical procedures. This technique uses barbed suture threads that are introduced under the skin, hoisting the dermis to create a lifted appearance. Those sutures may be nonabsorbable or absorbable ones. The nonabsorbable ones were short-lived in clinical application, as they lost FDA approval in 2007 due to serious complications associated with its use. However, in the daily practice of skin ultrasound, we still find patients with those nonabsorbable sutures. Currently, absorbable suture suspension is FDA approved and is being used to address ptotic skin located primarily in the midface, jawline, and neck areas. On ultrasound, suspension sutures appear as an echogenic linear image, formed by two parallel echogenic lines, usually located in the subcutaneous tissue. Nonabsorbable sutures produce posterior acoustic shadowing, while absorbable ones do not unless very-high-frequency probes are utilized as when a complication occurs.

Complications associated with thread-lifting technique include asymmetry, rippling and puckering, infection, granuloma, thread loss, and thread breakage. Ultrasound can be helpful in almost all complications, specially in identifying fluid surrounding the suture and inflammatory nodules and locating parts of thread after breakage [9].

9.3   Conclusion

Ultrasound has an important role in identifying cosmetic fillers and suspension sutures, as well as in the characterization of associated adverse effects, thus providing additional information to the clinical exam by guiding accurate therapeutic strategies.

References

1. Wortsman X. Identification and complications of cosmetic fillers: sonography first. J Ultrasound Med. 2015;34(7):1163–72.
2. Cheng LY, Sun XM, Tang MY, Jin R, Cui WG, Zhang YG. An update review on recent skin fillers. Plast Aesthet Res. 2016;3:92–9.
3. Berlin AL, Hussain M, Goldberg DJ. Calcium hydroxylapatite filler for facial rejuvenation: a histologic and immunohistochemical analysis. Dermatol Surg. 2008;34(Suppl 1):S64–7.
4. Alijotas-Reig J, Fernandez-Figueras MT, Puig L. Inflammatory, immune-mediated adverse reactions related to soft tissue dermal fillers. Semin Arthritis Rheum. 2013;43(2):241–58.
5. DeLorenzi C. Complications of injectable fillers, part 2: vascular complications. Aesthet Surg J. 2014;34(4):584–600.
6. da Aquino Cavallieri F, de Almeida Balassiano LK, de Bastos JT, da Fontoura GHM, de Almeida AT. Persistent, Intermittent Delayed Swelling PIDS intermittent swelling: late adverse reaction to Hyaluronic Acid fillers. Surg Cosmet Dermatol. 2017;9(3):218–22. https://doi.org/10.5935/scd1984-8773.201793931.
7. Pérez-Pérez L, García-Gavín J, Wortsman X, Santos-Briz Á. Delayed adverse subcutaneous reaction to a new family of hyaluronic acid dermal fillers with clinical, ultrasound, and histologic correlation. Dermatol Surg. 2017;43(4):605–8.
8. Quezada-Gaón N, Wortsman X. Ultrasound-guided hyaluronidase injection in cosmetic complications. J Eur Acad Dermatol Venereol. 2016;30:e39–40.
9. Ogilvie MP, Few JW Jr, Tomur SS, et al. Rejuvenating the face: an analysis of 100 absorbable suture suspension patients. Aesthet Surg J. 2018;38(6):654–63.

Podiatric Dermal Sonography

10

Richard Kushner and Robert L. Bard

A special chapter is devoted to these disorders since the foot is the ultimate and most uniquely human weight bearing structure where biomechanics play an important role in diagnosis and treatment. The causative factors of aberrant biomechanics create another clinical consideration in lesion formation and therapy of lower extremity disease.

Blood flow evaluation is a measure of inflammatory activity and tumor aggression and is covered elsewhere as is the physics of 3D image reconstruction with Doppler histogram analysis. Benign and malignant cutaneous disorders in previous chapters affect the foot and ankle, including the nail bed.

10.1 Vascular Tumors

Angiomas and similar benign tumors are better treated if the locoregional vasculature is mapped in the preop setting to anticipate potential complications. Vascular disease may be evaluated by blood flow Doppler analysis of the posterior tibial and pedal digital arteries.

Plaque may be observed as well as low or absent flow conditions (Fig. 10.1).

A hypovolemic region may be cyanotic casting a blue discoloration of a toe which may be mistaken for melanoma. This "blue toe" syndrome diffusely and homogenously discolors the entire nail bed and should not be easily confused with acral melanoma.

Certain verrucae (viral warts) may be vascular with a central vessel extending to the surface. Differentiating a wart from an amelanotic melanoma is due to the vertical Doppler flow commonly found in the benign lesion (simulating a tornado pattern) while the melanoma vascularity tends to be diffuse and horizontal in appearance (hurricane pattern).

10.2 Weight-Bearing Lesions

True bursae and potential or adventitial bursa are initiated and affected by chronic trauma. The subcutaneous lesions may form a subdermal mass and often produce dermal thickening and occasional discoloration (Fig. 10.2a, b).

Palmar and plantar skin is glabrous meaning hairless with a double-layered epidermis. Epidermal thickening over a joint is termed cornification or clavus, while the common callus is in other areas where intermittent pressure and

R. Kushner (✉)
Kushner Podiatry, New York, NY, USA

R. L. Bard
Director, The AngioFoundation, New York, NY, USA
e-mail: rbard@cancerscan.com;
www.angiofoundation.org

© Springer Nature Switzerland AG 2020
R. L. Bard (ed.), *Image Guided Dermatologic Treatments*,
https://doi.org/10.1007/978-3-030-29236-2_10

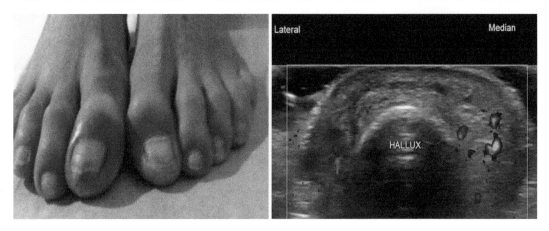

Fig. 10.1 Blood flow differentiates from low-flow disorder with incipient necrosis

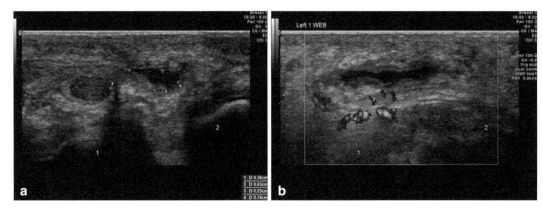

Fig. 10.2 Shearing force-induced inflamed bursal sac targeted for image-guided injection. (**a**) Transverse scan shows web space cystic area. (**b**) Doppler longitudinal scan demonstrates thick-walled bursal sac and hyperemia in underlying tendon

friction initiate a defense mechanism. Thickness of the epidermis may be demonstrated at high resolution alerting the podiatrist the safe depth limit for debridement procedures. While there are rare benign hyperkeratotic disorders of the epidermis, the thickening of the intraepidermal tissues appears as a black region that is differentiated from fluid by pressure application which shifts liquid content in real-time imaging. The dorsal layer of epidermal thickening often spares the underlying dermis (Fig. 10.3). Acute trauma may produce hemorrhagic areas which produce visible pigmentation in the epidermis. This callus is

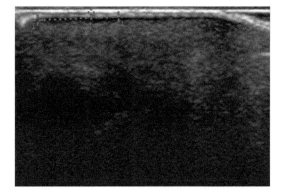

Fig. 10.3 Double-layered epidermis shows depth of callus-sparing dermis

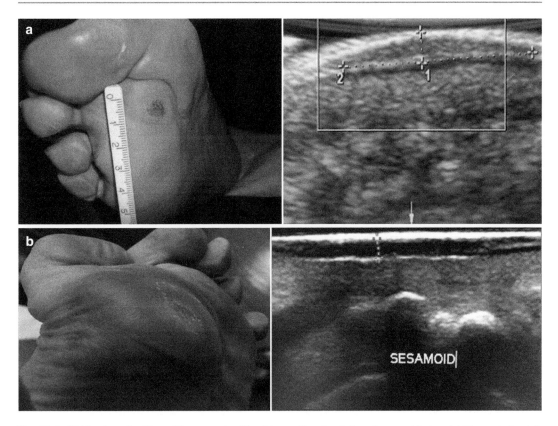

Fig. 10.4 Thickening of epidermal layer causing blood into callus simulating pigmented lesion. (**a**) Plantar lesion left sonogram right side. (**b**) Plantar region at sesamoid sonogram right side shows fractured sesamoid

exclusively situated between the dorsal and ventral epidermis (Fig. 10.4a).

The cause of callus formation may also be related to an underlying bone abnormality such as this fragmented tibial oriented sesamoid bone; thus the presence of thickened epidermal tissues should prompt the search for a causative process (Fig. 10.4b) [1–4].

Doppler imaging ruled out malignant vascularity as would the new optical technologies of OCT (optical coherence tomography) and RCM (reflectance confocal microscopy) that show surface vessels up to 1.5 mm in tissue depth. These technologies are discussed in other chapters and will probably have greater application in podiatry in the near future.

Rarely, chronic epidermal thickening will calcify and must be differentiated from subdermal calcinosis or calcinosis cutis (Fig. 10.5a) and crystal-forming diseases such as gout and CPDD or pseudogout (chronic pyrophosphate deposition disease) (Fig. 10.5b).

10.3   Cysts

The epidermal cyst (formerly called sebaceous cyst) is usually dermally located but extends to the epidermis with a tiny nipple or be wholly located in the subdermal recesses. While new cystic lesions are usually echo free, thin walled, and horizontally oriented, older cysts often contain echoes of debris, thick walls, and vertical orientation (Fig. 10.6).

Since a cystic focus appears as a subcutaneous region and may be hard and immobile if chronic, the differential diagnosis must include a bone lesion such as osteoma or, rarely, sarcoma or metastatic focus. Since the boney cortex is easily seen, a protrusion from the bone with intact bone outline and lack of cortical erosion ascertained, a radiographic investigation may be avoided (Fig. 10.7). Certain primary sarcomas and vascular metastases, such as breast cancer, melanoma, and renal cell carcinomas, may show hyperemia on Doppler blood flow imaging.

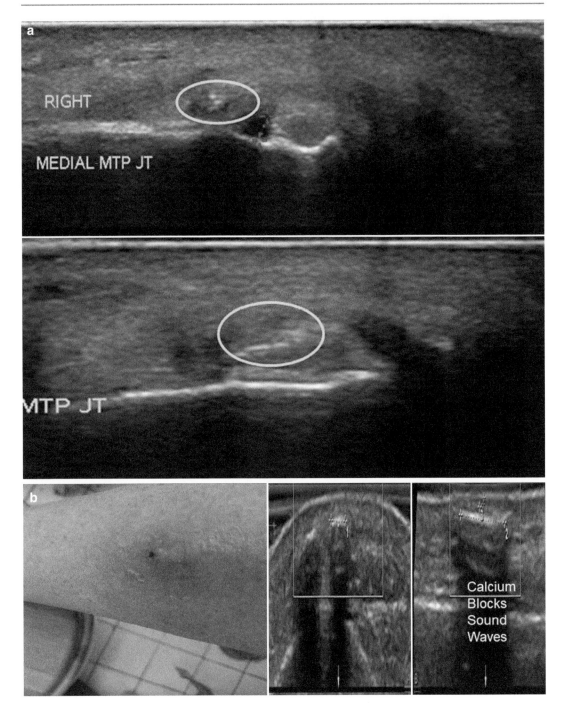

Fig. 10.5 (**a**) Calcinosis cutis-dermal or subdermal calcium may deflect or break needle. (**b**) Crystals from gout or CPDD may be differentiated from calcinosis cutis

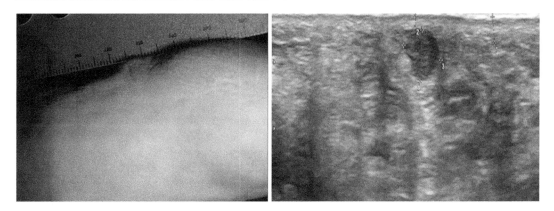

Fig. 10.6 Intradermal location differentiates cyst from scar due to inflammatory or foreign body reaction

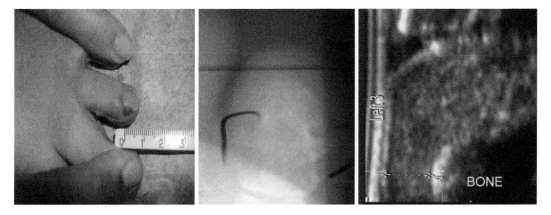

Fig. 10.7 Cortical intact outline differentiates benign osteoma from fracture or osteosarcoma

10.4   Foreign Bodies

Sonography is particularly important in the foot since both weight bearing and movement will affect the distribution in the affected region. The foreign body may fracture with displacement of fragments or be forced into locations unexpected by the initial portal of entry.

An intratendon location cannot be easily imaged during a surgical exploration, whereas sonography can pinpoint the site before or during surgery with intraoperative probes. Surgical image-guided foreign body removal has been performed by the US Army field surgeons for over 20 years with highly reduced surgical morbidity.

Foreign bodies that lie predominantly in the horizontal plane appear as linear bright echoes with or without the accompanying black shadow on standard 2D imaging. Since the 3D is multiplanar, the greatest dimension will be more easily identified in one of the three planes that occur simultaneously while scanning. A further refinement of 3D imaging is the 4D potential, which is real-time operator adjustment of the probe angle and position while scanning to optimize the foreign body in its most recognizable silhouette (Fig. 10.8). Note how the fiberglass thread is barely distinguishable from the normal nail bed structures on 2D but appears in stark contrast to the background in the 3D version. Splinter imaging is particularly optimized by the use of very high-frequency probes which can show the fragmented strands (Fig. 10.8a), perilesional fluid, and black sonic shadowing which may be missed by lower frequency probes (Fig. 10.8b). Significant perilesional fluid allows easier extraction of splinter and is better mapped at higher frequency potentially permitting minimally invasive removal by forceps.

Similarly, intraepidermal superficial splinters may appear as pigmented lesions to the naked eye but are quickly triangulated in depth by the 2D and 3D technology (Fig. 10.9). Subdermal lesions are likewise difficult to image in 2D; however the frequent occurrence of perilesional fluid due to local inflammatory processes creates a black background for the foreign object to be highlighted. In this case, the sea urchin spine remains uncalcified rendering radiographic imaging useless (Fig. 10.10). The foreign body may remain asymptomatic for prolonged periods or rapidly develop into complications including pain from abscess formation, chronic discharging wound with sinus tracts, necrotizing fasciitis, granulomas leading to bone and joint destruction including tendon infiltration with shredding and tearing, vascular events including thrombophlebitis with or without pulmonary emboli, and generalized massive soft tissue injury [5–12].

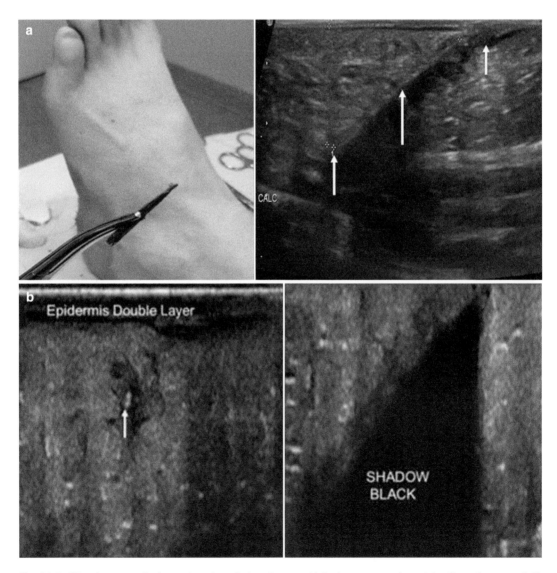

Fig. 10.8 3D volume permits better detection of glass fragment(s) in 4 cm square plane. (**a**) splinter fragment (left) sonogram (right) shows shadowing by subdermal fragment white arrows. (**b**) Transverse sonogram (L) shows cross section of splinter longitudinal sonogram shows full length as demonstrated by 3 cm shadow (R). (**c**) R image shows pigmented lesion L 2D and 3D sonogram

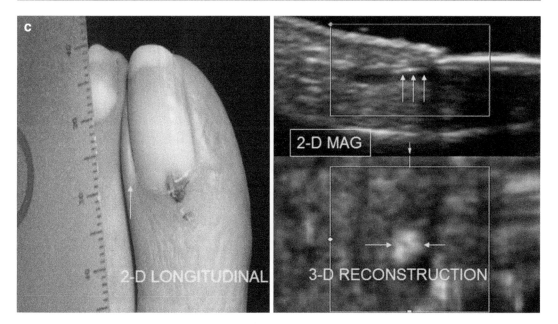

Fig. 10.8 (continued)

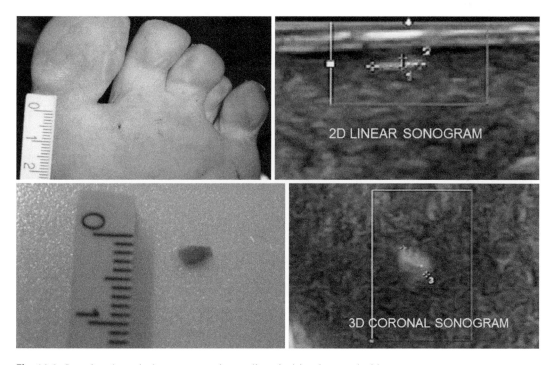

Fig. 10.9 Location above the basement membrane allows incisional removal without scar

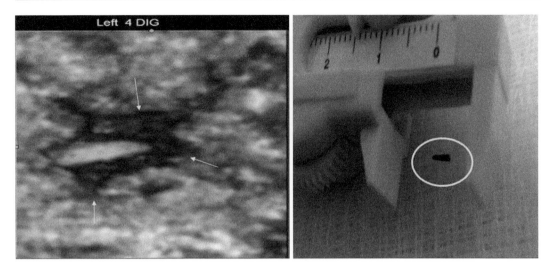

Fig. 10.10 Lack of Doppler flow suggests scarification a possible postop complication

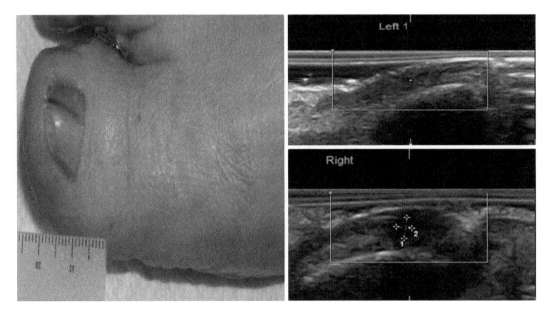

Fig. 10.11 Avascular granuloma differentiated from melanoma: note early cortical erosion

10.5 Inflammatory Lesions

Subungual granulomas produce dark inflammatory tissue reaction that stands out in the lighter nail bed tissues (Fig. 10.11). Long-standing lesions can erode the adjacent boney cortex and generate pigmented stripes or nail plate irregularities. Very-slow-growing tumors, including the glomus vascular lesion, often produce scalloping of the underlying bone that may be imaged without radiographs. Angiomatous areas may be associated with other findings such as epidermal thickening due to callus formation (Fig. 10.12) in this biopsy-proven hemangioma.

Chronic dermal inflammation in psoriasis, lupus erythematosus, and scleroderma including the growing list of connective tissue disorders with skin manifestations which may use sonography to guide treatment decisions. While epider-

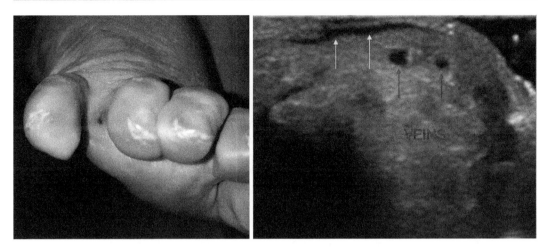

Fig. 10.12 Lesion avascularity rules against melanoma

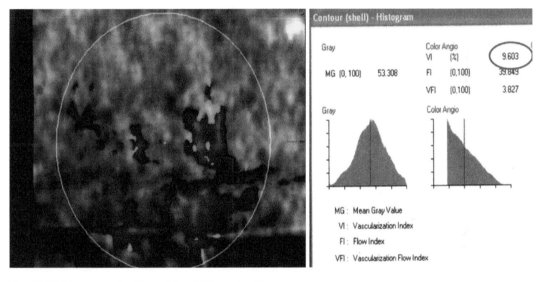

Fig. 10.13 Extravasated epidermal blood differentiated from nevus

mal and dermal depth changes are easily performed, the use of 3D Doppler histogram analysis allows a quantifiable marker to demonstrate treatment effectiveness. Since the degree of inflammation is proportional to the number of inflammatory vessels, the 3D measurement of vessel density in a given volume provides a baseline of the current inflammatory process, and serial scans produce a timeline of treatment change by measuring the vessel density index (VDI) which is expressed as a percentage of abnormal vessels in the region under investigation (Fig. 10.13) [13, 14].

Subdermal inflammation is now a common finding in cosmetic procedures and surgical interventions, and panniculitis may appear as dermal discoloration or irregularity. Note the dermal thickening and mottled echo pattern of the subcutaneous fat which is usually homogeneously dark. Trauma in the metatarsal region also produces this irregularity of the fatty tissues in the region of the hallux (Fig. 10.14).

Metatarsalgia associated with plantar plate degeneration or tearing is readily demonstrable by MRI or sonography; however, dynamic ultrasound allows the patient to point out the painful region that may be overshadowed by other findings on MRI such as neuromas or bursitis (Fig. 10.15).

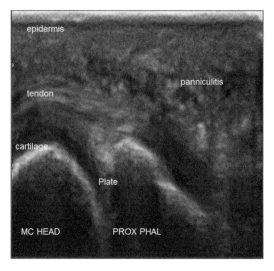

Fig. 10.14 Inflammation from filler injections which have a black box warning for injections on weight bearing areas

10.6 Melanoma

Given the deadly nature of acral melanoma, especially in the nail and sole of the foot, any pigmented lesion merits serious ultrasound Doppler investigation. While malignant melanoma is classically evaluated by the tumor depth (Breslow) or dermal layer invasion (Clark's level) and signs of surface ulceration, there exist better mechanisms for malignant tumor potential detection. Genetic expression testing and optical evaluation are being explored, but the vessel density index mentioned above in the inflammatory processes is a proven criterion that is currently used worldwide. Clearly the lack of dermal invasion and absence of neovascularity are indicative of a nonlethal disorder (Fig. 10.16) [15, 16].

3D Doppler histogram analysis is the optimal method of determining the malignant potential with a rapid noninvasive study. In the new milieu of oncoimmunologic treatments, the progression of therapy will be serially mapped by the 3D vessel density index to predict success or failure [17]. Alterations in vessel density occur earlier than

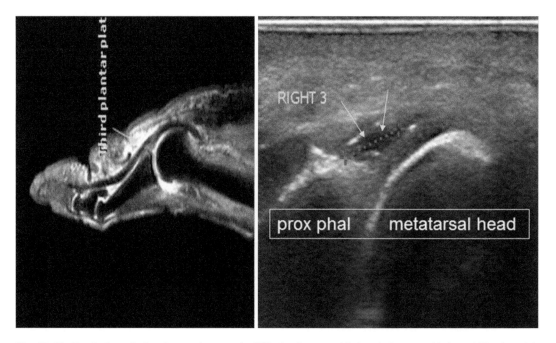

Fig. 10.15 Surgical repair for plantar plate tear is difficult—image-guided prolotherapy with immobilization aids treatment

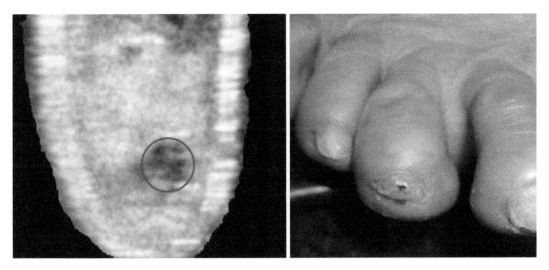

Fig. 10.16 Avascular pigmented lesion favors benign process in patients of color or without recall of injury

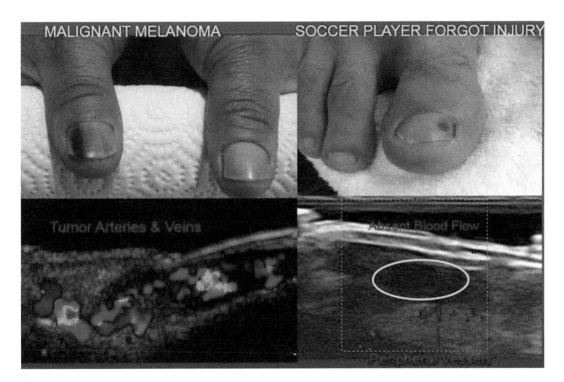

Fig. 10.17 Avascular lesion differentiated from hematoma and melanoma

visible or other non-Doppler imaging alterations. The possibility of a cancer's biologic nature changing or the tumor response to treatment diminishing can be quickly ascertained and evaluated allowing timely change in therapeutic options (Fig. 10.17).

References

1. Blechschmidt E. Die architecture de fersenpolsters. Morphologisches Jahrbuch. 1934;73:20–68.
2. Tietze A. Concerning the architectural structure of the connective tissue in the human sole. Foot Ankle. 1982;2:252–9.

3. Steiness IB. Vibratory perception in diabetes. Acta Med Scand. 1957;158:327–35.
4. Kim W, Voloshin AS. Role of the plantar fascia in the load bearing capacity of the human foot. J Biomech. 1995;28:1025–33.
5. Tantray MD, Rather A, Gull Y, et al. Role of ultrasound in detection of radiolucent foreign bodies in extremities. Surg Trauma Limb Reconstr. 2018;13(2):81–5.
6. Fakoor M. Prolonged retention of an intramedullary wooden foreign body. Pak J Med Sci. 2006; 22:78–9.
7. Freund EI, Weigl K. Foreign body granuloma: a cause of trigger thumb. J Hand Surg Br. 1984;9:210.
8. Choudhari KA, Muthu T, Tan MH. Progressive ulnar neuropathy caused by delayed migration of a foreign body. Br J Neurosurg. 2001;15:263–5.
9. Meurer WJ. Radial artery pseudoaneurysm caused by retained glass from hand laceration. Pediatr Emerg Care. 2009;25:255–7.
10. Flom LL. Ellis GL Radiologic evaluation of foreign bodies. Emerg Med Clin North Am. 1992;10:163–76.
11. Little CM, Parker MG, Callowich MC, et al. The ultrasonic detection of soft tissue foreign bodies. Invest Radiol. 1986;21:275–7.
12. Harcke TH. Sonographic localization and management of metallic fragments. Mil Med. 2012;177:988–92.
13. Mehta T, Raza S. Power Doppler sonography of breast cancer: does vascularity correlate with node status or lymphatic vascular invasion? Am J Roentgenol. 1999;173(2):303–7.
14. Merce LT, Alcazar J. Clinical usefulness of 3-dimensional sonography and power Doppler angiography for diagnosis of endometrial carcinoma. J Ultrasound Med. 2007;26:1279–87.
15. Lassau N, Spatz A. Avril MF et al Value of high frequency ultrasound for preoperative assessment of skin tumor. Radiographics. 1997;17:1559–65.
16. Wortsman X. Sonography of facial cutaneous basal cell carcinoma. J Ultrasound Med. 2013;32:567–72.
17. Lassau N, Chami L, Chebil M, et al. Dynamic contrast enhanced ultrasonography and anti-angiogenic treatments. Discov Med. 2011,11.18–24.

OCT-Guided Laser Treatment and Surgery

11

S. Schuh and J. Welzel

11.1 Introduction: OCT-Guided Treatment

Image-guided treatment is the future. In modern medicine imaging does play an essential part in the process of not only detecting and diagnosing diseases but also monitoring of therapy responses or disease progression and is extremely helpful during the treatment process.

Optical coherence tomography (OCT) is the device which fulfills these needs in the field of dermatology very well. Its use to aid with the diagnosis and decision upon the suitable therapy of non-melanoma skin cancer—towards more and more novel minimally invasive treatments, which require noninvasive imaging devices for diagnosis and therapy control—is already proven. Together with the technical development of the dynamic OCT (D-OCT), which enables the visualization of the vascularization of the skin and its tumors, D-OCT offers many possibilities for image-guided treatment such as OCT-guided laser treatment and surgery and allows for differentiation between different skin tumors and for decisions on optimal therapy for the patient.

11.2 OCT Technology

First of all, here are some technical details about OCT. It is a fast, noninvasive, in vivo imaging device, which was first applied by Huang et al. in 1991 in ophthalmology for the visualization of the retina [1]. In dermatology its use was first described by Welzel et al. in 1997 [2].

The technique of OCT is based on the principle of the Michelson interferometry. Light is split into a probe as well as a reference beam through a beam splitter. The probe beam is projected into the skin, whereas the reference beam is directed towards a reference mirror. The back-scattered light from the tissue as well as from the reference mirror interferes, if the light from both sides has the same optical way to the detector and the wavelengths correspond with each other within the coherence length of the light. The interference signal is then taken to create an image of the microstructures of the skin.

To clarify things, the term structural OCT will be used for all variants of OCT devices, which depict tissue structure, whereas the term dynamic OCT stands for structural OCT combined with an overlay of the vasculature. Structural OCT is already established as a useful tool for the diagnosis of non-melanoma skin cancer like basal cell carcinomas (BCC) [3–5]. BCC can be diagnosed with a high sensitivity (96%) and specificity (75%) due to characteristic criteria [3], for

S. Schuh (✉) · J. Welzel
Department of Dermatology, University Hospital Augsburg, Augsburg, Germany
e-mail: Sandra.Schuh@uk-augsburg.de

© Springer Nature Switzerland AG 2020
R. L. Bard (ed.), *Image Guided Dermatologic Treatments*,
https://doi.org/10.1007/978-3-030-29236-2_11

example, dark ovoid structures with a darker border within a bright stroma.

In the development process, there were different types of OCT devices available on the market. Generally, OCT has a higher image resolution and contrast but a lower penetration depth than ultrasound. One of the OCT machines was a high-definition OCT, which allowed a higher optical resolution but at the expense of a smaller field of view and a lower penetration depth. The latter, which allows the measurement of the tumor thickness, is necessary for treatment decision. Therefore, nowadays the OCT device in routine use provides an imaging depth of 1–2 mm and generates 2D and horizontal real-time images of some square millimeters of the skin without the use of a contrast agent. The imaging depth of the reflectance confocal microscopy (RCM) is a lot lower (<0.2 mm), despite the fact that RCM can discriminate single cells, which is not possible with OCT due to its resolution of 3–15 μm [6]. Moreover, OCT does not allow the visualization of fluorescent markers like RCM. OCT is best used for the architectural display of superficial structures of the skin, the epidermis and upper dermis including the papillary dermis and upper reticular dermis. The subcutis is typically not visible, just in very thin skin.

Nevertheless, with structural OCT it is not possible to diagnose melanoma certainly from dysplastic nevi. A new approach of OCT, the dynamic OCT, shows promising results to help with the differential diagnosis of melanocytic lesions [7]. It is a software-based technique that allows the detection of motion in the OCT images. The principle behind it is that from the same skin location, multiple OCT images were taken within a short time, and then the microscopic differences between the OCT images were evaluated. Due to this, the motion could be discriminated from the static tissue, which corresponds to blood flow. Thus, the specially adjusted software algorithm detects motion of particles due to blood flow. Therefore, a D-OCT image of the region of interest means the visualization of both the structural OCT, revealing the tissue structure, and the dynamic part, showing the vascular morphology of the blood vessels in this area. This method is also known as speckle-variance OCT [8], decorrelation-mapping OCT [9], optical microangiography [10], or OCT angi-

ography as well as dynamic OCT. There are two other methods that are comparable to D-OCT: Doppler OCT and laser speckle contrast imaging (LSCI). Doppler OCT can also detect blood flow in skin but with less sensitivity due to higher noise. However, the detection of motion is based on changes in intensity in Doppler OCT than in phase like in D-OCT [11, 12]. In addition to the very similar features of LSCI, D-OCT has a higher resolution, so that it is possible to resolve depth below skin and single fine blood vessels [13]. Blood flow can be detected between 0.1 and 1.0 mm/s; blood that is flowing slower like fluid in lymph vessels or static cannot be registered.

The images in this chapter were taken with a commercially available OCT scanner VivoSight Dx (Michelson Diagnostics Ltd, Maidstone, Kent, UK), equipped with D-OCT imaging software (see Fig. 11.1). The D-OCT was developed within the EU-funded project called ADVANCE "Automatic Detection of Vascular Networks for Cancer Evaluation" Grant No. 621015. The image resolution (7.5 μm in the lateral and 5 μm in the axial direction) is enough to show details of the vertical skin morphology and blood capillaries, but not for single cells. The field of view is 6 mm × 6 mm and the penetration depth is 1–2 mm, but the D-OCT algorithm has a limit of 0.5 mm. At a higher imaging depth, there is too much background noise, which interferes with the signal. Moreover, the flexible handheld probe carries a color video camera to allow the exact positioning on a region of interest and shows an overview image. For the imaging process, there is no need for gel or for other previous preparation of the skin before the simple measurement. Besides, the OCT system uses a laser with a near infrared wavelength (1300 nm) to operate. One scan is generated in 15 s for structural OCT resp. and 30 s for D-OCT and contains a 3D block (6 mm × 6 mm × 2 mm) of 120 D-OCT images with a pixel size of 4.3 μm over the field of view. The vertical and horizontal images can then be analyzed separately at the same time at any requested depth. For this cause the so-called fitted en face view is helpful, too. This tool allows the automatic fitting of the image plane to the skin surface, so that the skin surface topography could be followed without disruption along with all structures like blood vessels below the

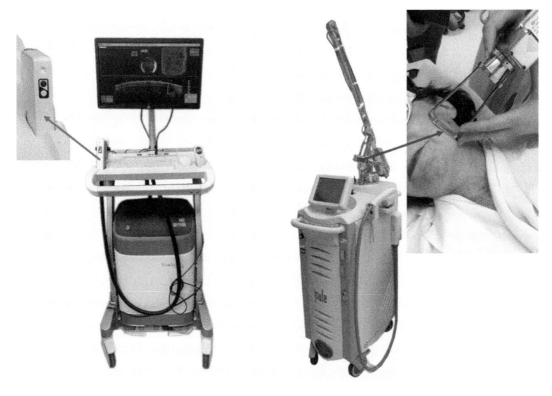

Fig. 11.1 OCT device VivoSight Dx with the white button (multi-slice scan) and the black button (free-run mode) and the Sciton laser with a special handpiece designed for OCT-guided laser therapy of BCC, the BCC Scanner

skin. For the dynamic evaluation, blood vessels are shown with a red overlay, which varies in brightness according to the strength of the blood flow, on top of the structural gray tissue image.

OCT—in addition with the dynamic software algorithm for the detection of vascular changes—is therefore a technically very qualified tool to play an important role, not only in the diagnosis of skin pathologies but equally important in the image-guided treatment of diseases.

11.3 Indications of OCT-Guided Treatment

11.3.1 Margin Mapping of BCC Using OCT During Mohs Micrographic Surgery

11.3.1.1 Summary

Mohs micrographic surgery (MMS) is the first-line treatment for high-risk BCC, meaning high risk of relapse, recurrent BCC, and those on a delicate location [14, 15]. OCT is a helpful noninvasive device to diagnose BCC. Thus, the application of OCT for the outline of the tumor margins before MMS may significantly decrease the number of surgical steps and offer a lot of advantages to patients and the health system.

11.3.1.2 Background

BCC is the most common skin cancer in the Caucasian population, and its incidence is permanently increasing [16]. Despite the fact that BCC grow slowly, the tumors can extend destructively, and without proper therapy, there is a high risk of relapse. Even if surgery is the preferred therapeutic approach for BCC, recurrences occur frequently. The reasons are mainly based on the histologic subtype (fibrosing, micronodular, or basosquamous) but also the location (midface or around the orifices) matters. For this reason, a complete removal of the tumor avoiding unnecessary excision of healthy skin along with maximally possible function integrity of the affected skin area and the best cosmetic outcome is the main goal.

This purpose is most likely achieved with MMS, which consists of at least two surgical steps. The first part is the excision of the tumor and after that the histopathological examination of the margins under a microscope for the absence of tumor. In the second step, there is always another surgery, either the wound closure if there was reported tumor clearance of the margins or further excisions until all tumor tissue is removed along the borders and in the last case, then finally the closure of the defect could follow. To conduct MMS, financial, time- and resource-related aspects need to be considered as well as high professional skills of the surgeons are necessary, since MMS is time consuming and requires possibly multiple surgical interventions [17]. This is also the cause why MMS is not uncomplicated and why a patient in a poor general condition won't maybe be able to undergo MMS.

This is the moment when OCT comes into play. OCT is already established in the diagnosis of BCC like several studies have proven, and furthermore the subtype and the tumor depth could be assessed with it [3, 18–21]. Therefore, OCT can aid to determine the lateral borders of BCC prior to MMS like a pre-histological examination of the tumor. At the moment the surgeon is not aware of the actual tumor spread. According to MMS standards, the extent of the lesion is investigated clinically or dermoscopically, and then a 2 mm safety distance is added. In this case, when tumor borders are exactly determined by OCT and excised at the same marking, OCT can not only enhance the rate of complete BCC excision—meaning tumor free margins within only one step of surgery—but also at the same time reduce the wound size and perhaps consequently lead to a smaller suture, a smaller scar, and finally a better cosmetic outcome. In a wider context, when multicenter studies prove that OCT can significantly decrease the number of surgical steps, clinics, practices, and hospitals are able to treat more patients more effectively with OCT-guided MMS.

11.3.1.3 Procedure

At the University Hospital of Augsburg in the dermatological department, we conducted a preliminary trial from October to December 2015 [22]. The approval of the Institutional Review Board has been obtained. The aim of this study was to find out if and maybe how many steps of MMS could be quantitatively reduced with OCT image-guided margin mapping. Ten patients were measured to map the borders of the BCC with OCT before surgery. An ongoing study with two groups, each consisting of 50 patients, one with standard MMS and one with OCT-guided MMS, is expected to prove again the key results from the preliminary study of 2015.

All tumors were photographed with the photo camera Sony Cybershot (16.1 mega pixels, 5× optical zoom), and dermoscopic images were taken with the dermoscope Dermlite HR (3Gen, S. Juan Capistrano, CA, USA). The OCT scans for the mapping of the BCC were all created with the VivoSight DX from Michelson Diagnostics (described above) (Fig. 11.1). The borders were determined with a silver permanent marker (Edding® 780 creative 0.8 mm in silver color), which proved to show the best image results after testing [22]. When the OCT scans over the silver-marked margin, the pen leaves a hyper-reflective thin line with an underlying dark shadow (Fig. 11.2). This shadow separates the inner center with the BCC from the hopefully tumor-free area around it.

The whole OCT image-guided margin mapping consists of five steps. First the visible outline of the tumor was traced clinically with the help of the dermoscope (Fig. 11.2). Additionally to this contour, the safety distance was enhanced about 2 mm. Then the first OCT measurement was done in the center of the lesion as a multislice scan (white button) (Fig. 11.3). Thus, the diagnosis can be confirmed, the structures (like nodules, cysts) and the subtype can be assessed, and the tumor thickness can be measured from the epidermis to the lowest border of the BCC. To ensure good quality, calm measurement is essential. If there are crusts on top of the lesion, a scan

Fig. 11.2 First step: clinical and dermoscopical outline of the tumor with 2 mm safety distance with a pre-surgical marker (silver-inked pen), which is visible in OCT as a shadow (green arrow)

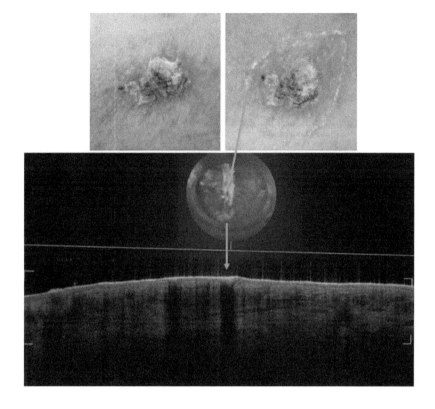

Fig. 11.3 Second step: center OCT scan of the lesion as a multi-slice scan (white button on OCT device) to confirm the diagnosis, assess the structures and the subtype, as well as measure the tumor thickness. In this case it is a nodular cystic BCC (red asterisks). Cross-sectional view 6 mm × 2 mm

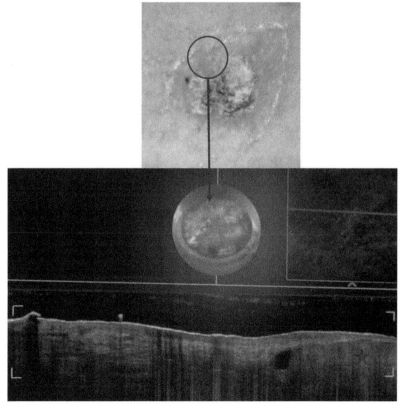

Fig. 11.4 Third step: OCT margin mapping in free-run-mode (black button on OCT device) clockwise (starting at 12 o'clock) with a small overlap along the previously clinically and dermoscopically marked borders (blue circles). As a guide the silver-inked margin should always be in the middle of the color video camera (green arrow). Dark ovoid tumor nodules are visible in the OCT image inside and outside of the border (red arrows). Cross-sectional view 6 mm × 2 mm

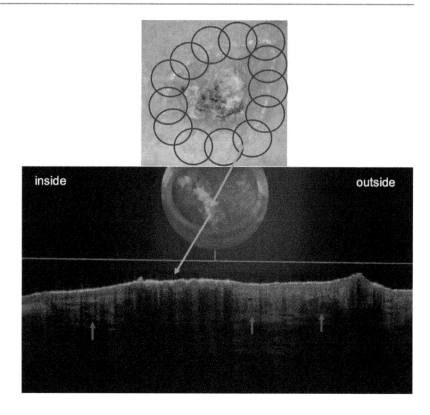

from the side should be made, since measurements through the crust are not possible and lead to dark artifacts (Fig. 11.3). The evaluation of the OCT scan is mainly done when looking at the transversal images, but sometimes the en face view can be of help, too. In the third step, the actual margin mapping process is performed. Scans are conducted in free-run-mode (black button) and clockwise (starting at 12 o'clock) with a small overlap along the previously clinically and dermoscopically marked borders (Fig. 11.4). For orientation, the silver-inked margin should always be positioned in the center of the color video camera. Then the scan was performed from the BCC affected area across the pen-marked border to the maybe healthy skin. The pen mark represents an optical landmark for the demarcation or extension of the margins. In step four the border is extended preserving a safety distance of 2 mm, if BCC residuals are found outside the initial margin in the same OCT-guided border mapping procedure (Fig. 11.5). After the assurance that there is no

suspect area for BCC outside of the silver border, the silver marking should be traced with a regular surgical marker, and then the final and fifth step is MMS based on the OCT-defined margins (Fig. 11.6).

After the excision on the outermost borders of the lesion and the marking of the tissue with different colors, the center, basis, and all margins were separately examined in the histology lab with "Tübinger Torte" technique (Fig. 11.6).

A video (https://www.youtube.com/watch?v= CUUanxi-LdM) filmed, cut together and edited by Lawrence da Silva from Michelson Diagnostics, shows the practical demonstration of the OCT margin mapping procedure and can provide more information about it.

11.3.1.4 Findings and Benefits

The results of this preliminary trail showed that 8 of 10 BCC clinical margins were correctly mapped using OCT and led to a complete excision in one surgery. Two of 10 BCC did not catch every tumor cell even with OCT mapping,

Fig. 11.5 Fourth step: extension of the borders, if BCC residuals are outside the original margin, preserving a safety distance of 2 mm. When margins are tumor-free in OCT, the patient is ready for surgery. The red circle indicates a small longish tumor island in between two silver-inked margins (green arrows in clinical and dermoscopic image). Cross-sectional view 6 mm × 2 mm

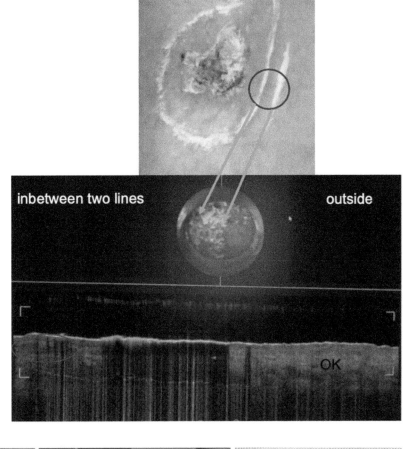

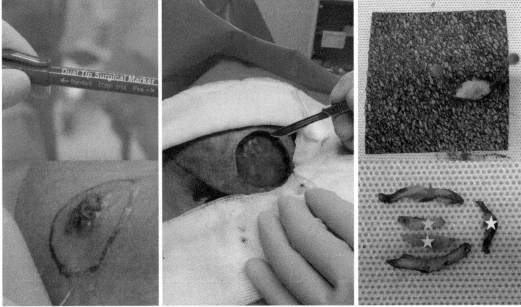

Fig. 11.6 Fifth step: trace of the silver marking with a regular surgical marker. MMS based on the OCT-defined margins. Tissue was marked with different colors for orientation. Then all parts, the center (green asterisks), the lateral margins (red asterisks), and the bottom (yellow asterisk) were separately examined using "Tübinger Torte" technique

because of a higher tumor thickness and an infiltrative subtype. Other imaging limitations are bleeding tumors, crusts, and difficult to access locations like inner eye corner or nasal wings. Still, the results indicate and what hopefully the bigger study will prove that a decrease in the average MMS steps from 1.7 to 1.2 should be possible [22]. This fact is in accordance with other findings [23–27]. Less MMS stages also mean a shorter overnight hospital stay for the patient. The reduction of MMS stages could also be a financial benefit for the clinic, practice, or hospital performing MMS. Due to less MMS stages per patient, more patients could be treated per week, leading to a higher reimbursement income rate and reducing waiting time for MMS. Besides, the average size of the wound defect would be smaller, leading to a smaller and hopefully cosmetically more appealing scar with preserved functional capacity. Moreover, the OCT-guided MMS requires less time for the whole procedure, saving MMS stages, but of course OCT mapping time needs to be considered, which is about 15–20 min per lesion.

Apart from that, OCT might also be useful at the first patient's visit and not only before MMS. With OCT the BCC could be evaluated in advance. For example, OCT could assess, if clearly outlined BCC are possible to be excised by simple surgery, if poorly demarcated BCC need MMS, or if alternative therapy like topical treatment could be applied. OCT can also help to predict the number of MMS steps that will be necessary, which could also help the patient to plan the down-time before the hospital stay and the dermatology facility to organize the surgery schedule.

11.3.2 Dynamic OCT of Skin Tumors: Blood Vessel Patterns of BCC, AK, Bowen's Disease, and Invasive SCC Help with the Diagnosis

11.3.2.1 Summary

Before starting a treatment of a skin tumor, the diagnosis should be correctly made. Since many noninvasive treatments are nowadays available for non-melanoma skin cancer, the demand for noninvasive devices for diagnosis is high, because a punch biopsy along with a scar just for diagnosis, and especially in cosmetically sensitive areas, is not what is desired if the patient could be treated noninvasively. Therefore, the use of D-OCT and the possibility to look at blood vessel patterns allows a distinction between the non-melanoma skin cancer types and could help sort out the lesions for excision, type of excision (simple, MMS), or noninvasive treatment, to allow a more precise, effective, and individual patient-oriented therapy.

11.3.2.2 Basal Cell Carcinoma

Despite the fact that many morphological features of BCC were detected in structural OCT, just a few studies evaluated the chance of OCT to differentiate BCC subtypes, which were more or less successful [28–34]. One recent study showed that the differentiation between BCC subtypes is possible if both structural and dynamic OCT features are considered [35]. Why is the discrimination between BCC subtypes necessary? Depending on the subtype, the treatment will be chosen differently, for example, as for superficial BCC noninvasive treatment is possible, whereas for infiltrative BCC MMS excision is the safest option. With that knowledge the BCC and therefore the patient could get the best suitable, individual treatment. Even the punch biopsy, which only reflects one part of the lesion, but which is still the gold standard for diagnosis, could miss the main part of the subtype if the BCC consists of more than one subtype. With OCT the whole structural overview of the tumor can be pictured, and therefore also the dominant subtype can be evaluated. D-OCT offers the possibility to investigate the superficial, the so-called telangiectasias, which are also visible in dermoscopy, and deeper blood vessels, which are depicted as extended vertical vessel columns in cross-sectional images. In general, more vessels and a chaotic formation of small to very large vessels can be noticed at the site of the BCC compared to healthy adjacent skin in the en face images [36].

With that in mind, Themstrup et al. analyzed structural and dynamic characteristics [35].

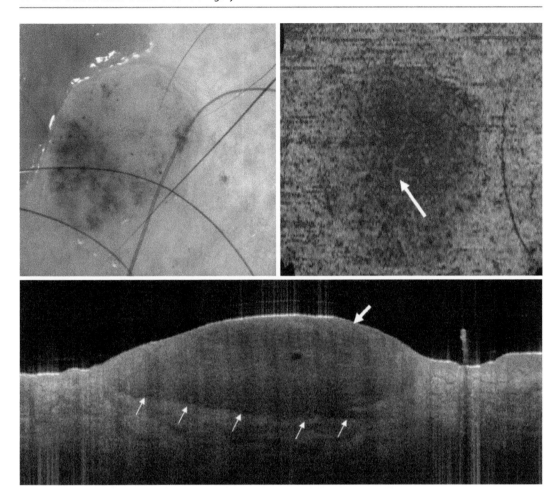

Fig. 11.7 Dermoscopic image and cross-sectional OCT scan (6 mm × 2 mm) of a nodular BCC on the back as a sharply outlined ovoid hyporeflective structure (thin white arrows) with a bright surrounding stroma and a local thin-ner epidermis (thick white arrow). Serpiginous vessels in branching shape forming an outlined figure can be seen in D-OCT (en face view 6 mm × 6 mm)

For the nodular BCC, sharply outlined ovoid hyporeflective structures with a bright surrounding stroma were a significant diagnostic criterium compared to the other two subtypes [35] (Fig. 11.7). A circumscribed thinner epidermis next to these dark features indicated also an increased risk for nodular BCC [35] (see Fig. 11.7). When looking at the vessels, the presence of serpiginous vessels, branching structures, and vessels forming an outlined figure was found in nodular BCC significantly more frequent in comparison with the other two BCC forms [35] (Fig. 11.7).

This is in contrast with superficial BCC. If serpiginous or branching vessels were apparent, the risk of the subtype being superficial was significantly reduced [35]. No major vessel pattern was specific for superficial BCC. However, superficial BCC showed significantly more small hyporeflective ovoid nests protruding from the epidermis than nodular or infiltrative BCC [35] (Fig. 11.8).

Infiltrative BCC are more difficult to diagnose. If narrow elongated dark structures appear in the OCT image, like a "shoal of fish," then this is a hint for an infiltrative BCC (Fig. 11.9). To diagnose the infiltrative subtype, what cannot be seen is more important than what can be seen in the OCT picture. Dark rims at the borders of the round dark structures were signifi-

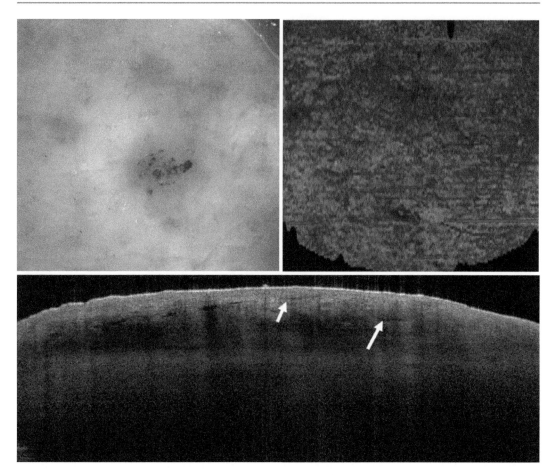

Fig. 11.8 Dermoscopic image and cross-sectional OCT scan (6 mm × 2 mm) of a superficial BCC on the back. Small hyporeflective ovoid protrusions (thick white arrows) from the epidermis are visible. No major vessel pattern is typical for superficial BCC in D-OCT (en face view 6 mm × 6 mm)

cantly less displaying infiltrative BCC than the other two subtypes [35]. Highly present lines significantly reduced the risk of the presence of an infiltrative BCC [35].

These findings may aid to make more informed individual patient-oriented decisions in case of a BCC treatment. But sometimes when performing an OCT scan, it happens that the pink lesion that is measured does not show typical BCC criteria. Then other non-melanoma skin cancer forms or even an amelanotic melanoma need to be considered.

11.3.2.3 Actinic Keratosis, Bowen's Disease, and Invasive Squamous Cell Carcinoma

To start with the precancerous lesions, in structural OCT actinic keratoses (AK) can be recognized when there is a thick stratum corneum and epidermis, but each of the layers can be very well differentiated, which also accounts for the dermoepidermal junction (DEJ) as a dark layer in between epidermis and dermis (Fig. 11.10). The hyperkeratosis as well as its reflection varies, depending on the degree and form of the AK. The

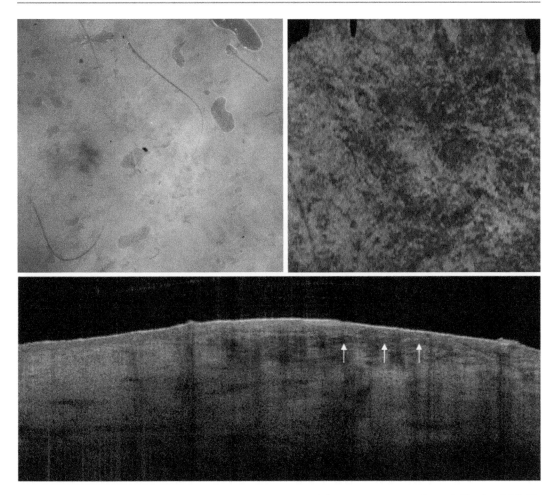

Fig. 11.9 Dermoscopic image and cross-sectional OCT scan (6 mm × 2 mm) of an infiltrative BCC on the leg. Narrow elongated dark structures like a "shoal of fish" (thin white arrows) are a hint for an infiltrative BCC. No major vessel pattern is typical for infiltrative BCC in D-OCT (en face view 6 mm × 6 mm)

hyperkeratosis is also the one to blame why AK, Bowen's disease, and SCC are sometimes hard to differentiate, because the artifacts due to the scales cause shadows and impede the evaluation of the DEJ as well as a look into deeper skin layers. Nevertheless, hyperkeratotic AK are more hyper-reflective, whereas some AK appear hyporeflective because of parakeratosis [36]. In D-OCT Themstrup et al. show that there is one typical vessel pattern for AK, which proved to be statistically significant: the curves of the vessels [37]. A small number of blobs can be found in 55–77% of AK and also lines [37]. The vascular pattern "mesh" is characteristically observed in AK at 300 μm [37] (Fig. 11.10).

Moreover, Bowen's disease or squamous cell carcinoma (SCC) in situ exhibits more or less the same structural OCT features than AK, just with fewer or no hyperkeratosis (Fig. 11.11). In D-OCT in one-third of Bowen's disease, the high number of blobs at 300 μm differed significantly from the presence in AK or SCC [37], whereas curves were mainly absent. At 300 μm the typical vessel pattern was "mottle" in Bowen's disease [37] (Fig. 11.11).

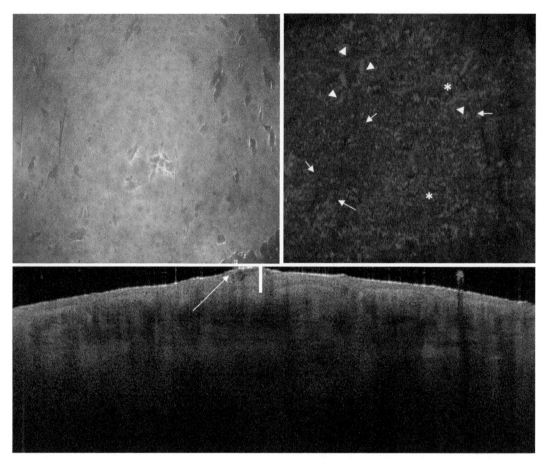

Fig. 11.10 Dermoscopic image and cross-sectional OCT scan (6 mm × 2 mm) of an actinic keratosis (AK) on the forehead. A thickened stratum corneum (thin white arrow) and epidermis are visible and easy to discriminate (thick white bar). The horizontal D-OCT image (6 mm × 6 mm) shows the typical vessel pattern for AK, the curves of the vessels (white arrowhead), but also a small number of blobs (white asterisk) and lines (white arrow) can be found. The vascular pattern "mesh" is characteristically observed in AK at 300 µm

In structural OCT invasive SCC are sometimes difficult to diagnose. Features like the conversion or disruption of the normal skin layers like the DEJ and the dermis can also be found in some lesions of AK or Bowen's disease (Fig. 11.12). As a sign of invasion, the protrusions from the epidermis into the dermis can occur in different forms and with several shades of reflectivity [36]. However, in SCC the main vessel type is lines. A few blobs were visible, too [37] (Fig. 11.12). The characteristic vessel pattern for SCC was "chaos" in relation to AK and Bowen's disease [37]. Investigations of the vessel diameter proved that there are significantly bigger vessels present in SCC than in healthy skin. The same accounts for vessel density in relation to normal skin as well as to the precancerous lesions, which was for both groups only statistically significant at 150 µm [37] (Fig. 11.12).

11.3.2.4 Conclusion

To sum up, together, structural and dynamic OCT, can provide more information about the present lesion for the correct diagnosis and

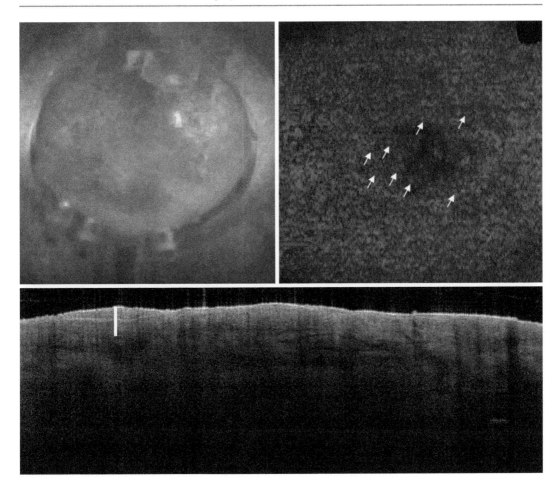

Fig. 11.11 Dermoscopic image and cross-sectional OCT scan (6 mm × 2 mm) of Bowen's disease on the forehead. Bowen's disease also shows a thickening of the stratum corneum and epidermis (thick white bar). In the horizontal D-OCT image (6 mm × 6 mm), a high number of blobs (white arrow) is present. At 300 µm the typical vessel pattern is "mottle" in Bowen's disease

therefore help to discriminate the different types of non-melanoma skin cancer but also the BCC subtypes, as well as to guide the physician in his or her decision about the best suitable therapy.

11.3.3 OCT-Guided Laser Therapy

11.3.3.1 Summary

Besides OCT-guided surgery, OCT could also aid in the investigation of the efficacy and safety of laser treatments. Until now there is no evidence of the actual impact laser treatment has on the skin and what kind of changes it causes deep down in the skin after the removal of different lesions, depending on ablative, fractional, or a coagulating Nd:YAG laser therapy. OCT can provide an insight into the skin and show the evolving processes after laser therapy either to confirm successful treatment response or to help find the right laser settings for the individual lesion. Nd:YAG laser therapy is one of the approved treatment options for BCC. In this case OCT has the potential to demonstrate the BCC criteria, which influence the treatment response. Moreover, OCT can also help to detect recurrences early in the course of time.

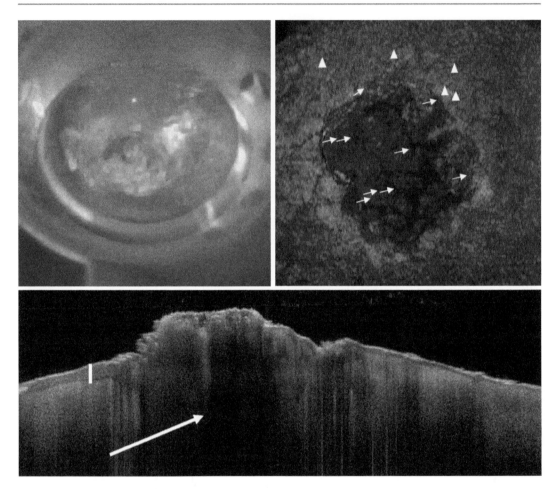

Fig. 11.12 Dermoscopic image and cross-sectional OCT scan (6 mm × 2 mm) of squamous cell carcinoma (SCC) on the right hand. Disruption of normal skin layers (thick white bar) like the DEJ and the dermis can be registered as well as the protrusions from the epidermis into the dermis (thick white arrow). In the horizontal D-OCT image (6 mm × 6 mm), the main vessel type is lines (thin white arrows); a few blobs (white arrowhead) were visible, too. The characteristic vessel pattern for SCC is "chaos." Vessel diameters are bigger in SCC than in healthy skin, and vessel density is higher in relation to normal skin

11.3.3.2 OCT-Guided Laser Treatment of BCC

According to the current treatment guideline for BCC, Nd:YAG laser therapy is one of the therapeutic options. Nd:YAG laser therapy is a coagulation laser, which destroys tumor blood vessels. A recently published small study by Ortiz et al. with 31 BCC showed a high response rate (90%) without leaving a scar [38]. The diagnosis and follow-up were done by punch biopsy. One disadvantage of all noninvasive treatments is the missing histological reassurance. Thus, for every noninvasive therapy, clinical or histological follow-up is recommended. OCT, which can diagnose even clinically unclear BCC with a sensitivity of 95%, a specificity of 75%, and an accuracy of 87% [39], is also able to do the follow-up in the course of time to detect BCC recurrences early but can help even more in advance of the treatment. For example, the measurement of the tumor thickness, the determination of the subtype, and the evaluation of the tumor vessels are important aspects that have an impact on the treatment response.

The study by Ortiz et al. showed no serious side effects, but the efficacy of an OCT-guided laser therapy has not been evaluated until now. In the context of a bigger ongoing study, the preliminary trial should be confirmed and proved to see if the OCT-guided Nd:YAG laser therapy is an efficient and safe procedure for the removal of BCC, so that surgery or topical therapy can be avoided. Moreover, it should be examined if OCT is a helpful tool to select suitable BCC for laser therapy (with features like a tumor thickness less than 1.2 mm, a specific subtype, dense network of blood vessels, topography of tumor vessels). At the same time, it can be investigated if the use of OCT allows a better evaluation of the laser therapeutic efficacy than clinical and dermoscopic evaluation alone. Besides, the study should prove if OCT can follow up the treatment response noninvasively and detect BCC relapses early. In this case it can be analyzed if and to what extent BCC recurrences during OCT follow-up correlate with histological BCC relapses. Furthermore the cosmetic outcome of the

Nd:YAG laser therapy will be documented and evaluated. It should be examined if and to what extent side effects and pain occur. Patients' and doctor's assessment of the laser therapy is recorded. One aim is also to investigate if there is a connection between BCC subtype, tumor thickness, tumor blood vessels, and efficacy of the laser therapy.

At last, these OCT parameters can then be used to modify the settings of the Nd:YAG laser (energy density, spot size, pulse duration) in a following study and therefore to increase the efficacy of the treatment.

First descriptive results show an immediate visible response of the BCC after Nd:YAG laser treatment with OCT (Sciton Laser, Sciton Inc., Palo Alto, California, US, BCC Scanner, 140 J/cm², 10 ms, temperature (N/A, 10 pulses needed). This representative example OCT image (but also dermoscopy) illustrates that immediately after the therapy the tumor is kind of "cooked" (white area

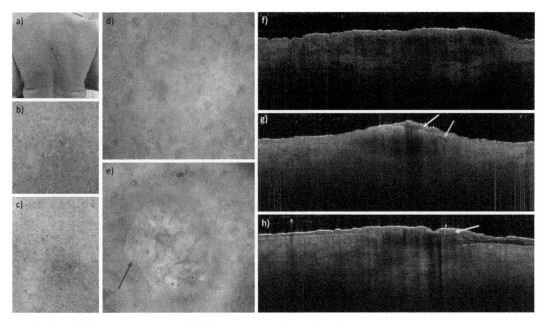

Fig. 11.13 Clinical, dermoscopic, and OCT images of a nodular BCC, TD 0.73 mm on the back before and right after resp. one week after the Nd:YAG laser treatment. (**a, b, d**) show the clinical and dermoscopic images of the BCC on the back before and (**c, e**) right after laser therapy. The OCT image in (**f**) depicts the BCC before, (**g**) right after, and (**h**) after one week of laser therapy (cross-sec-

tional view 6 mm × 2 mm). Immediately after the therapy, the tumor is kind of "cooked" (white area, see red arrow in (**e**)) and gets necrotic (see green arrow in **g**). The epidermis and dermis appear blurrier compared to the OCT scan before (**f**) vs. (**g**), and right after therapy there is already the occurrence of crusts (see (**g, h**))

in dermoscopy) and gets necrotic (Fig. 11.13). The whole tumor, including epidermal and dermal parts, appear blurrier compared to the previous OCT scan before. Sometimes right after laser treatment, a blister is also visible (Fig. 11.14). There can also be slight bleeding, leakage of serous fluid, and already some occurrence of crusts. Right after treatment the blood vessels are less dense compared to the OCT scan taken before therapy (Fig. 11.14). After one week the BCC area is covered with scales and crusts, which makes it harder to evaluate the scan, but the primary results indicate that despite that fact OCT can already depict tumor clearance or BCC residuals (Fig. 11.15). BCC recurrence then shows areas which weren't treated sufficiently or strong enough.

Therefore, OCT allows for the first time to look at the changes laser therapy really causes deep in the skin and can help to guide more effective laser treatment of BCC.

11.3.3.3 OCT-Guided Laser Treatment of Vascular Lesions, Lentigines, and Others

Besides OCT-guided laser treatment of BCC, OCT can observe the alterations other laser treatments cause, for example, ablative, fractional, or laser therapy of vascular lesions.

One example is the treatment of a telangiectasia on the left hand before broad band light (BBL) treatment (Sciton Laser, Sciton Inc., Palo Alto, California, US, parameters: 560 filter, 20–22 J/cm^2, 20 ms, 15 °C, round adapter, 4 pulses needed) (Fig. 11.16). The dermoscopic, clinical, and D-OCT image show immediate changes right after BBL therapy. When looking at the clinical image as well as in dermoscopy, the color of the telangiectasia is lighter. The dermoscopic picture also indicates that the vessels are not as sharply demarcated as before. The appearance is fuzzier. There was also a decreased capillary refill. The

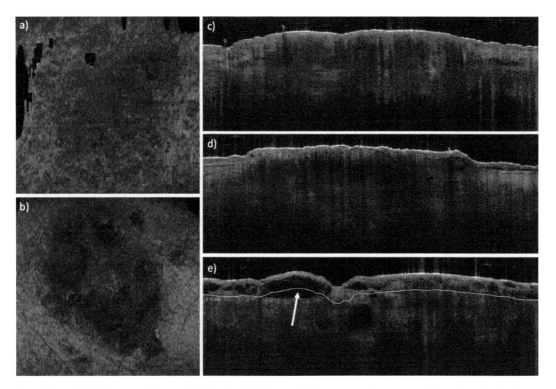

Fig. 11.14 D-OCT images of the same BCC in Fig. 11.13 before (**a**, **c**), right after (**b**, **e**), and one week after (**d**) Nd:YAG laser therapy. Blood vessels appear less dense, and the structural surface seems rougher after 1 week (**c** vs. **d**). Sometimes blisters are visible directly after laser therapy (white arrows in **e**). En face view at a depth of 300 μm, 6 mm × 6 mm, cross-sectional view 6 mm × 2 mm

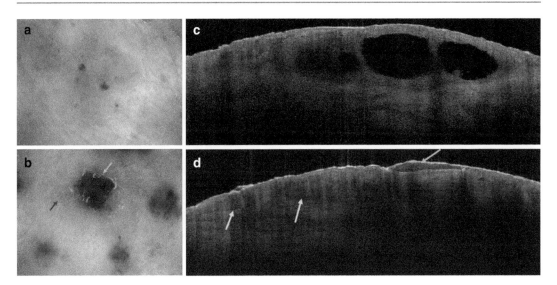

Fig. 11.15 Dermoscopic and OCT images of a nodular BCC, TD 1.0 mm on the lower right back before (**a**, **c**) and one week after (**b**, **d**) Nd:YAG laser therapy. Scales and crusts (green arrow in **b**, orange arrow in **d**) as well as BCC residuals (red arrow in **b**, yellow arrows in **d**) can be seen in the OCT picture (cross-sectional view 6 mm × 2 mm). Even in dermoscopy the original BCC telangiectasias are still visible (see red arrow in **b**)

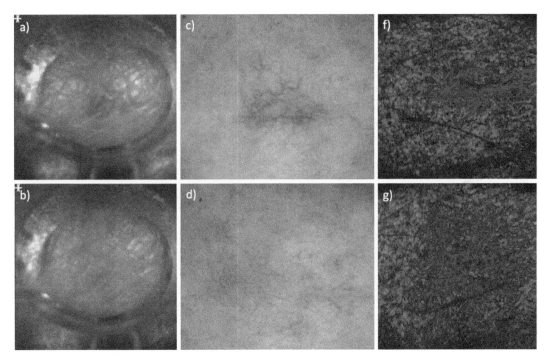

Fig. 11.16 Telangiectasia on the left hand before (**a**, **c**, **f**) and after (**b**, **d**, **g**) broad band light (BBL) treatment. The clinical (**b**) and dermoscopic (**d**) images show a lighter color than before (**a**, **c**). In dermoscopy the vessels are not as sharply demarcated and fuzzier as prior to the therapy. The D-OCT ((**f**) en face view at a depth of 300 μm, 6 mm × 6 mm) image before therapy depicts vessels of a bigger caliber and afterwards (**g**) multiple smaller to very small blood vessels are visible, even in the surroundings of the former telangiectasia

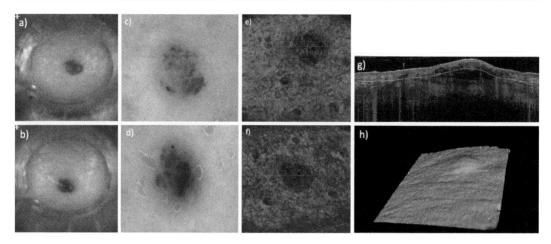

Fig. 11.17 An angioma on the chest before (**a, c, e, g, h**) and after Nd:YAG laser therapy (**b, d, f**). Before the treatment the slightly elevated vascular lesion (**e, g, h**) shows the clustered vessel network inside of the angioma. After therapy a color change from light red (**a, c**) to dark red until brown occurred (**b, d**) is visible. In the horizontal D-OCT, the former clustered vessel network is now occluded, and the angioma shows a thrombosis of the vessels (**f**)

D-OCT image reveals that the vessels of a bigger caliber are gone and are now replaced by multiple smaller to very small blood vessels, even in the surroundings of the former telangiectasia.

A vascular lesion like a cherry angioma on the right chest is another case of successful Nd:YAG laser therapy (Sciton Laser, Sciton Inc., Palo Alto, California, US, parameters: 1064 nm, 3 mm single spot, 2 shots of 80 J/cm², 60 ms, temperature (N/A), 2 shots of 100 J/cm², 60 ms, temperature (N/A), without cooling, 4 pulses needed) (Fig. 11.17). Before the treatment the slightly elevated vascular lesion shows the clustered vessel network inside of the angioma. After the two first shots of Nd:YAG laser at 80 J/cm², the clinical and dermoscopic image did not show any change. After another two shots of 100 J/cm², a color change from light red to dark red until brown occurred. In the horizontal D-OCT image, there is the confirmation of the effect. The former clustered vessel network is now occluded, and the angioma shows a thrombosis of the vessels.

Another lesion, an age spot on the right dorsal wrist, was treated with Er:YAG laser therapy (Sciton Laser, Sciton Inc., Palo Alto, California, US, parameters: 2940 nm, 3 pulses should give a total of 90 microns depth, 4 mm single spot, 30 μm set, 1.0 Hz, temperature (N/A), 3 pulses needed) (Fig. 11.18). The clinical and the dermoscopic images indicate that the former pigmented lesion is gone, but there is an increase of blood vessels, leading to an erythema, which is clearly visible. In the horizontal OCT image, the ablation zone can be seen. The structural OCT image gives proof of the desired laser depth of 90 μm. An ablation of the entire epidermis can be noticed.

Moreover, fractional Er:YAG laser therapy was applied on a healthy left forearm (Sciton Laser, Sciton Inc., Palo Alto, California, US, parameters: 2940 nm, 110 μm depth at 11% density, ProFractional handpiece used) (Fig. 11.19). The laser spots obviously left traces clinically and dermoscopically as well as in the horizontal and cross-sectional OCT image. The formerly adjusted depth of 110 μm could be confirmed with OCT. Each laser spot was 110 μm deep.

11.3.3.4 Conclusion

These were some examples for different types of laser therapy. With the use of OCT, the laser treatments could be checked on their efficacy, on the changes, which the lasers evoked in the skin tissue, and on the vasculature. It helps to under-

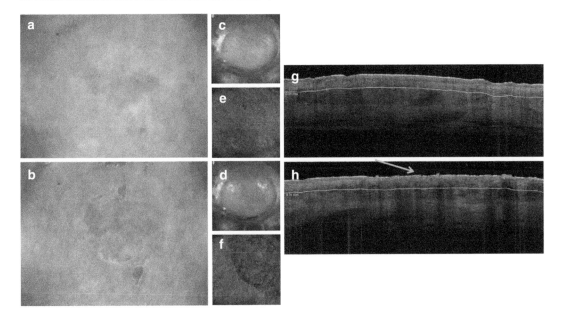

Fig. 11.18 Age spot on the right dorsal wrist before (**a**, **c**, **e**, **g**) and after (**b**, **d**, **f**, **h**) treatment with Er:YAG laser therapy. The clinical (**c**, **d**) and the dermoscopic images (**a**, **b**) indicate that the former pigmented lesion is gone, but there is an increase of blood vessels, leading to an ery-thema, which is clearly visible in **b** and **d**. In the horizontal OCT image, there is the ablation zone after laser therapy (**f**) compared to before (**e**). The structural OCT image gives proof of the desired laser depth of 90 μm. An ablation of the entire epidermis can be noticed (orange arrow)

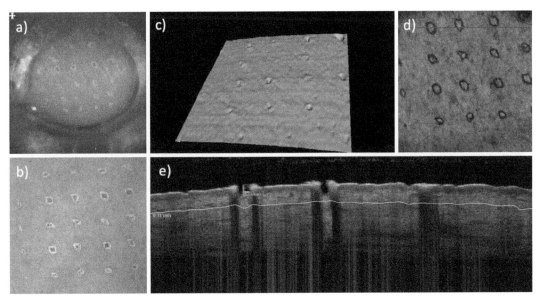

Fig. 11.19 Healthy left forearm after Er:YAG laser therapy. The laser spots obviously left traces clinically (**a**) and dermoscopically (**b**) and in the horizontal (**c**, **d**) and cross-sectional OCT image (**e**). The formerly adjusted depth of 110 μm could be confirmed with OCT (**e**)

stand and revise the processes that are going on and which possibly need to be adapted, if the treatment is not sufficient enough like in the case of the angioma or also for BCC laser therapy. There are many more possible indications for OCT-guided treatment conceivable, which need to be pursued, because with the help of OCT individual, patient-orientated efficient modern medicine is feasible.

11.4 Outlook

In modern medicine technology is playing a more and more important role. In former times dermatological treatments were conducted, because it has been done like that for years and no one asked how the goal of a good treatment response was achieved. Now OCT allows us to take a look into the skin, to perform a more efficient therapy, but also to prove a good or bad treatment outcome. And if it turns out that the therapy was not as good as expected, to maybe find out the causes that led to that experience. Despite the fact that knowledge skills in OCT are required, but which can be learned, technology like OCT makes the life of a physician easier and him or her more confident to provide the best possible medicine to his or her patient at present time. Innovations like handheld OCT or Line-field OCT (a combination of OCT and confocal microscopy) will perhaps be the next step in this direction [40, 41].

Overall it should be noted that OCT is more than just a tool for imaging. It is a clinical device for image-guided treatment which is the future of modern dermatologic medical practice.

References

1. Huang D, Swanson EA, Lin CP, Schuman JS, Stinson WG, Chang W, Hee MR, Flotte T, Gregory K, Puliafito CA, Fujimoto JG. Optical coherence tomography. Science. 1991;254(5035):1178–81.
2. Welzel J, Lankenau EM, Birngruber R, Engelhardt R. Optical coherence tomography of the human skin. J Am Acad Dermatol. 1997;37(6):958–63.
3. Ulrich M, Braunmuehl T, Kurzen H, Dirschka T, Kellner C, Sattler EC, Berking C, Welzel J, Reinhold

U. The sensitivity and specificity of optical coherence tomography for the assisted diagnosis of nonpigmented basal cell carcinoma: an observational study. Br J Dermatol. 2015;173(2):428–35.
4. Cheng HM, Guitera P. Systematic review of optical coherence tomography usage in the diagnosis and management of basal cell carcinoma. Br J Dermatol. 2015;173(6):1371–80.
5. Markowitz O, Schwartz M, Feldman E, Bienenfeld A, Bieber AK, Ellis J, Alapati U, Lebwohl MG, Siegel DM. Evaluation of optical coherence tomography as a means of identifying earlier stage basal cell carcinomas while reducing the use of diagnostic biopsy. J Clin Aesthet Dermatol. 2015;8(10):14–20.
6. Longo C, Pellacani G. Reflectance confocal microscopy. In: Katsambas AD, Lotti TM, Dessinioti C, D'Erme AM, editors. European handbook of dermatological treatments. 3rd ed. Berlin: Springer; 2015. p. 1129–37.
7. De Carvalho N, Welzel J, Schuh S, Themstrup L, Ulrich M, Jemec GBE, Holmes J, Kaleci S, Chester J, Bigi L, Ciardo S, Pellacani G. The vascular morphology of melanoma is related to Breslow index: an in vivo study with dynamic optical coherence tomography. Exp Dermatol. 2018;27(11):1280–6.
8. Mariampillai A, Standish BA, Moriyama EH, Khurana M, Munce NR, Leung MK, Jiang J, Cable A, Wilson BC, Vitkin IA, Yang VX. Speckle variance detection of microvasculature using swept-source optical coherence tomography. Opt Lett. 2008;33(13):1530–2.
9. Jonathan E, Enfield J, Leahy MJ. Correlation mapping method for generating microcirculation morphology from optical coherence tomography (OCT) intensity images. J Biophotonics. 2011;4(9):583–7.
10. An L, Qin J, Wang RK. Ultrahigh sensitive optical microangiography for in vivo imaging of microcirculations within human skin tissue beds. Opt Express. 2010;18(8):8220–8.
11. Zhao Y, Chen Z, Saxer C, Shen Q, Xiang S, de Boer JF, Nelson JS. Doppler standard deviation imaging for clinical monitoring of in vivo human skin blood flow. Opt Lett. 2000;25(18):1358–60.
12. Ren H, Ding Z, Zhao Y, Miao J, Nelson JS, Chen Z. Phase-resolved functional optical coherence tomography: simultaneous imaging of in situ tissue structure, blood flow velocity, standard deviation, birefringence, and Stokes vectors in human skin. Opt Lett. 2002;27(19):1702–4.
13. Boas DA, Dunn AK. Laser speckle contrast imaging in biomedical optics. J Biomed Opt. 2010;15(1):011109.
14. Schreiber MM, Moon TE, Fox SH, Davidson J. The risk of developing subsequent nonmelanoma skin cancers. J Am Acad Dermatol. 1990;23(6 Pt 1):1114–8.
15. Ad HTF, et al. AAD/ACMS/ASDSA/ASMS 2012 appropriate use criteria for Mohs micrographic surgery: a report of the American Academy of Dermatology, American College of Mohs Surgery, American Society for Dermatologic Surgery

Association, and the American Society for Mohs Surgery. J Am Acad Dermatol. 2012;67(4): 531–50.

16. Bath-Hextall F, Leonardi-Bee J, Smith C, Meal A, Hubbard R. Trends in incidence of skin basal cell carcinoma. Additional evidence from a UK primary care database study. Int J Cancer. 2007;121(9):2105–8.

17. Marzuka AG, Book SE. Basal cell carcinoma: pathogenesis, epidemiology, clinical features, diagnosis, histopathology, and management. Yale J Biol Med. 2015;88(2):167–79.

18. Sattler E, Kästle R, Welzel J. Optical coherence tomography in dermatology. J Biomed Opt. 2013;18(6):061224.

19. Olmedo JM, Warschaw KE, Schmitt JM, Swanson DL. Correlation of thickness of basal cell carcinoma by optical coherence tomography in vivo and routine histologic findings: a pilot study. Dermatol Surg. 2007;33(4):421–5.. discussion 425–426.

20. Olmedo JM, Warschaw KE, Schmitt JM, Swanson DL. Optical coherence tomography for the characterization of basal cell carcinoma in vivo: a pilot study. J Am Acad Dermatol. 2006;55(3):408–12.

21. Wahrlich C, Alawi SA, Batz S, Fluhr JW, Lademann J, Ulrich M. Assessment of a scoring system for Basal Cell Carcinoma with multi-beam optical coherence tomography. J Eur Acad Dermatol Venereol. 2015;29(8):1562–9.

22. De Carvalho N, Schuh S, Kindermann N, Kästle R, Holmes J, Welzel J. Optical coherence tomography for margin definition of basal cell carcinoma before micrographic surgery-recommendations regarding the marking and scanning technique. Skin Res Technol. 2018;24(1):145–51.

23. Pomerantz R, Zell D, McKenzie G, Siegel DM. Optical coherence tomography used as a modality to delineate basal cell carcinoma prior to Mohs micrographic surgery. Case Rep Dermatol. 2011;3(3):212–8.

24. RBRVS US Medicare Claims Database American Medical Association; 2011. Available at: www.ama-assn.org. Accessed: 1 Dec 2017.

25. Chan CS, Rohrer TE. Optical coherence tomography and its role in Mohs micrographic surgery: a case report. Case Rep Dermatol. 2012;4(3):269–74.

26. Wang KX, Meekings A, Fluhr JW, McKenzie G, Lee DA, Fisher J, Markowitz O, Siegel DM. Optical coherence tomography-based optimization of mohs micrographic surgery of Basal cell carcinoma: a pilot study. Dermatol Surg. 2013;39(4):627–33.

27. Alawi SA, Kuck M, Wahrlich C, Batz S, McKenzie G, Fluhr JW, Lademann J, Ulrich M. Optical coherence tomography for presurgical margin assessment of non-melanoma skin cancer—a practical approach. Exp Dermatol. 2013;22(8):547–51.

28. Boone MA, Suppa M, Pellacani G, Marneffe A, Miyamoto M, Alarcon I, Ruini C, Hofmann-Wellenhof R, Malvehy J, Jemec GB, Del Marmol V. High-definition optical coherence tomography algorithm for discrimination of basal cell carcinoma from clinical BCC imitators and differentiation between common subtypes. J Eur Acad Dermatol Venereol. 2015;29(9):1771–80.

29. Meekings A, Utz S, Ulrich M, Bienenfeld A, Nandanan N, Fisher J, McKenzie G, Siegel DM, Feldman E, Markowitz O. Differentiation of basal cell carcinoma subtypes in multi-beam swept source optical coherence tomography (MSS-OCT). J Drugs Dermatol. 2016;15(5):545–50.

30. Cheng HM, Lo S, Scolyer R, Meekings A, Carlos G, Guitera P. Accuracy of optical coherence tomography for the diagnosis of superficial basal cell carcinoma: a prospective, consecutive, cohort study of 168 cases. Br J Dermatol. 2016;175(6):1290–300.

31. von Braunmühl T, Hartmann D, Tietze JK, Cekovic D, Kunte C, Ruzicka T, Berking C, Sattler EC. Morphologic features of basal cell carcinoma using the en-face mode in frequency domain optical coherence tomography. J Eur Acad Dermatol Venereol. 2016;30(11):1919–25.

32. Maier T, Braun-Falco M, Hinz T, Schmid-Wendtner MH, Ruzicka T, Berking C. Morphology of basal cell carcinoma in high definition optical coherence tomography: en-face and slice imaging mode, and comparison with histology. J Eur Acad Dermatol Venereol. 2013;27(1):e97–104.

33. Boone MA, Norrenberg S, Jemec GBE, Del Marmol V. Imaging of basal cell carcinoma by high-definition optical coherence tomography: histomorphological correlation. A pilot study. Br J Dermatol. 2012;167(4):856–64.

34. Gambichler T, Plura I, Kampilafkos P, Valavanis K, Sand M, Bechara FG, Stücker M. Histopathological correlates of basal cell carcinoma in the slice and en face imaging modes of high-definition optical coherence tomography. Br J Dermatol. 2014;170(6):1358–61.

35. Themstrup L, De Carvalho N, Nielsen SM, Olsen J, Ciardo S, Schuh S, Nørnberg BM, Welzel J, Ulrich M, Pellacani G, Jemec GBE. In vivo differentiation of common basal cell carcinoma subtypes by microvascular and structural imaging using dynamic optical coherence tomography. Exp Dermatol. 2018;27(2):156–65.

36. Schuh S, Holmes J, Ulrich M, Themstrup L, Jemec GBE, Pellacani G, Welzel J. Imaging blood vessel morphology in skin: dynamic optical coherence tomography as a novel potential diagnostic tool in dermatology. Dermatol Ther (Heidelb). 2017;7(2):187–202.

37. Themstrup L, Pellacani G, Welzel J, Holmes J, Jemec GBE, Ulrich M. In vivo microvascular imaging of cutaneous actinic keratosis, Bowen's disease and squamous cell carcinoma using dynamic optical coherence tomography. J Eur Acad Dermatol Venereol. 2017;31(10):1655–62.

38. Ortiz AE, Anderson RR, DiGiorgio C, Jiang SIB, Shafiq F, Avram MM. An expanded study of long-pulsed 1064 nm Nd:YAG laser treatment of basal cell carcinoma. Lasers Surg Med. 2018;50(7):727–31.

39. Holmes J, von Braunmühl T, Berking C, Sattler E, Ulrich M, Reinhold U, Kurzen H, Dirschka T, Kellner C, Schuh S, Welzel J. Optical coherence tomography of basal cell carcinoma: influence of location, subtype, observer variability and image quality on diagnostic performance. Br J Dermatol. 2018;178(5):1102–10.

40. ITRI Taiwan; 2018. Available at http://www.oct-news.org/articles/8309812/handheld-skin-quality-optical-coherence-tomography/. Accessed 2 Dec 2018.

41. Dubois A, Levecq O, Azimani H, Siret D, Barut A, Suppa M, del Marmol V, Malvehy J, Cinotti E, Rubegni P, Perrot JL. Line-field confocal optical coherence tomography for high-resolution non-invasive imaging of skin tumors. J Biomed Opt. 2018;23(10):106007.

Reflectance Confocal Microscopy for the Diagnosis and Management of Skin Diseases

12

Radhika Srivastava, Catherine Reilly, and Babar Rao

12.1 Introduction

In vivo Reflectance Confocal Microscopy (RCM) is a noninvasive imaging modality that is used for the diagnosis of many dermatologic conditions.

12.1.1 History

The confocal microscope was initially conceptualized by Marvin Minsky in 1957 [1], and with advances in optical and electronic technology, the first confocal microscopes for skin imaging were developed in the late 1990s [2]. Lucid Inc. (Caliber ID, Rochester, New York, USA) released several commercially available confocal microscopes for skin imaging in 1997, including the VivaScope 1500 and VivaScope 3000. In 2007, the company launched VivaNet (Caliber ID, Rochester, New York, USA), a secure Health Insurance Portability and Accountability Act (HIPAA) compliant network online to facilitate image transfer, evaluation, and diagnosis. Most recently, in 2016, the US Centers for Medicare and Medicaid Services (CMS) granted RCM imaging of skin category I current procedural terminology (CPT) reimbursement codes [3].

RCM has expanded considerably in the past few decades, with growing interest from and by dermatologists, pathologists, and patients.

12.1.2 Optical System and Image Acquisition

Reflectance confocal microscopy utilizes an 830nm monochromatic laser to direct 22 mW of light into the skin. The light first travels to a beam splitter and further to an objective lens. The various structures of the skin have different indices of refraction, causing the light to be reflected back to the objective lens of the microscope. Once the light returns to the scope, it travels through a detector aperture, which collects only high-resolution signals, and creates the confocal image that is presented on the monitor [4]. Due to the different indices of refraction of cellular structures, some appear bright, such as keratin, melanin, and collagen, while others appear dark, generating the black and white confocal image [5].

There are currently two reflectance confocal microscopes that are commercially available. The VivaScope 1500 captures high-quality images and is preferred when the imaging flat surfaces. A drop of crystal plus white mineral oil which has a refractive index of 1.47, similar to that of the stratum corneum, is placed directly on the lesion. A square-shaped window with peripheral adhesive is directly attached to the patient's skin.

R. Srivastava (✉) · C. Reilly · B. Rao
Center for Dermatology, Rutgers Robert Wood Johnson Medical School, Somerset, NJ, USA
e-mail: rs1063@rwjms.rutgers.edu;
clarkcat@sas.upenn.edu

© Springer Nature Switzerland AG 2020
R. L. Bard (ed.), *Image Guided Dermatologic Treatments*,
https://doi.org/10.1007/978-3-030-29236-2_12

The window isolates an 8 mm × 8 mm surface area and ensures the scope remains in place during the procedure. Ultrasound transmission gel is added to the outward-facing side of the window, and the head of the scope is attached to the window.

Various imaging options are available, including block images, stacked images, and live video. The block images capture X–Y area within the window at different Z-depths and have the highest resolution. The Z-depth can be adjusted, up to approximately 200–300 μm below the skin's surface. Stack images isolate a specific 0.5 mm × 0.5 mm area of the skin and captures a series of images at increasing Z-depth. For example, the machine can capture up to 127 images at increasing 1.5 μm depth for one specific region. Finally, live video is available if observing the live movement of cellular structures is desired.

The VivaScope 3000 is an alternate device, often referred to as the "handheld." This scope is preferred for challenging locations, where attaching the square window required for the VivaScope 1500 may be difficult. Such areas may include cartilaginous surfaces like the nose and ears or mucosal surfaces like the lips and labia. Imaging preparation for the two scopes is similar, except the VivaScope 3000 has a circular window that lacks adhesive to attach to a set area of the skin. This allows for full range of motion while imaging. Stacked and single-stacked images 0.75 mm × 0.75 mm may be captured with the handheld device, as well as live video.

12.2 Image Interpretation and Clinical Applications

To evaluate RCM images, a systematic examination of each layer of skin is required: the epidermis, the dermoepidermal junction, and the dermis. The characteristics of normal skin on RCM are described in Table 12.1 [6, 7]. There is variation in the thickness of the skin layers and density of the adnexal structures based on age and the anatomical site. Familiarization with the appearance of normal skin facilitates recognition of atypical patterns and features associated with disease (Fig. 12.1).

Table 12.1 Reflectance confocal microscopy features of normal skin

Skin layer	RCM features
Epidermis	– Honeycomb pattern—a grid of well-demarcated polygonal keratinocytes – Dermatoglyphs (skin folds), hair shafts, follicular orifices, and eccrine ducts – Cobblestone pattern—aggregates of small polygonal cells with bright cytoplasm separated by less refractive outline, at the stratum basalis
Dermoepidermal junction	– Ringed-edged pattern—small bright cells surrounding dark-appearing ovoid dermal papillae
Dermis	– Blood vessels—round or canalicular dark spaces in which occasionally small bright cells, representing inflammatory cells, can be visualized – Collagen—bright elongated fibrillar structures arranged in a reticular pattern – Infundibula of the hair follicles can be visualized

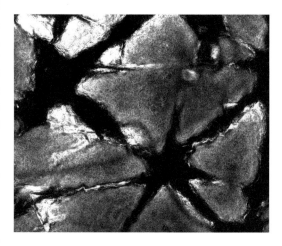

Fig. 12.1 Reflectance confocal microscopy of normal skin shows regular honeycomb pattern of the epidermis and visible dermatoglyphs

12.2.1 Melanocytic Neoplasms

RCM is well suited for the evaluation of melanocytic lesions, as melanin is highly refractile and has strong contrast on RCM imaging. Several scoring systems and algorithms that rely on the identification of benign and atypical features have been developed for the diagnosis of melanocytic lesions (Table 12.2) [8–10]. Benign patterns include the honeycomb pattern and cobble stone pattern at the epidermis (Fig. 12.2) and the ringed pattern (Fig. 12.3), meshwork pattern, and clod pattern at the dermoepidermal junction. Atypical features include pagetoid spread of bright atypical nucleated round-, dendritic-, or spindle-shaped cells in the epidermis (Fig. 12.4),

Table 12.2 Reflectance confocal microscopy features of melanocytic lesions

RCM feature	Description
Pagetoid spread	Cells with dark nuclei and bright cytoplasm in the superficial epidermis, may be round or dendritic, variable degree of atypia and pleiomorphism, may occupy variable surface areas of lesion
Ringed pattern	Bright rings at the dermoepidermal junction comprised of small bright cells surrounding dark dermal papilla
Meshwork pattern	Junctional thickenings at the dermoepidermal junction
Clod pattern	Large round dense compact nests of melanocytes at the dermoepidermal junction
Edged papilla	Dermal papilla with well-circumscribed contours
Non-edged papilla	Dermal papillae are not clearly outlined
Architectural disarray	Loss of normal architecture of the dermoepidermal, may be mild, moderate, or severe
Nest	Oval to round bright aggregate with well-defined borders comprised of frequently large and highly refractive cells
Junctional nest	Nests connected with epidermal basal layer that bulge into dermal papillae, may have variable shape and size, may have non-homogenous cellularity
Dermal nest	Nests below/not in direct connection with basal cell layer
Atypical cells at the dermoepidermal junction	Well-demarcated, round or dendritic cells with bright cytoplasm and dark nucleus, variable degree of atypia and pleiomorphism, may occupy variable surface areas of lesion

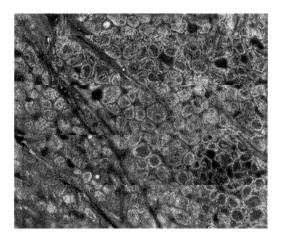

Fig. 12.2 Reflectance confocal microscopy of a benign nevus shows cobblestone pattern

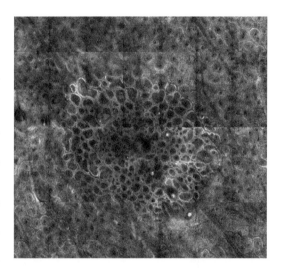

Fig. 12.3 Reflectance confocal microscopy of benign nevus shows the ringed pattern

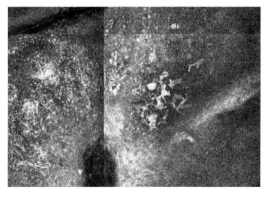

Fig. 12.4 Reflectance confocal microscopy of a melanoma shows large bright atypical dendritic cells in the epidermis

non-edged papilla and architectural disarray at
the dermoepidermal junction, and atypical cells
in a sheet-like distribution or forming irregular
nests in the dermis.

Benign nevi consist of one or a mix of the
benign patterns with the notable lack of atypical
features (Fig. 12.5) [11]. Junctional nevi are associated with the ringed pattern, compound nevi are
associated with the ringed pattern or the meshwork pattern, and intradermal nevi are associated
the clod pattern [12]. Dysplastic nevi are characterized by the presence of mostly benign features
and one to two atypical cytological or architectural features (Fig. 12.6) [11]. Histopathologic
features and grading of dysplastic nevi correspond well with RCM [11]. Melanomas are associated with the presence of greater than two to
three atypical cytological and architectural features (Fig. 12.7) [8]. Lentigo maligna and lentigo maligna melanoma display similar atypical
features RCM and with follicular localization of
atypical cells [13].

RCM has demonstrated consistently high
accuracy in the diagnosis of melanocytic lesions,
with a sensitivity of 93–100% and a specificity

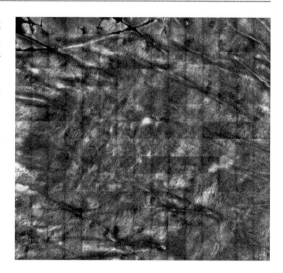

Fig. 12.6 Reflectance confocal microscopy of a dysplastic nevus with atypical meshwork pattern, round and dendritic atypical cells, and broadened junctional nests

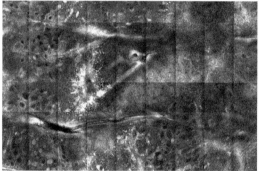

Fig. 12.7 Reflectance confocal microscopy of melanoma
shows large bright round and dendritic cells with severe
cytologic atypia

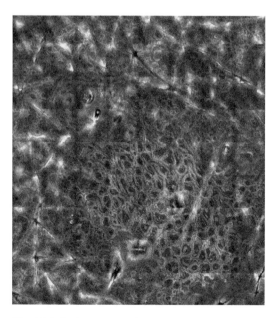

Fig. 12.5 Reflectance confocal microscopy of a benign
nevus shows a meshwork pattern and dermal and junctional nests, with no evidence of cellular or architectural
atypia

of 75–99% [14–17]. RCM is particularly useful
in the evaluation of clinically or dermoscopically
equivocal lesions as RCM has greater specificity
than dermoscopy [18, 19]. The high specificity
of RCM reduces the benign to malignant ratio of
biopsies from 18:1 with clinical judgement, 4:1
with dermoscopy, to 2.13:1 [20]. RCM is also
very useful in cases of hypomelanotic and amelanotic melanoma that may appear banal on clinical
and dermoscopic evaluation [21]. The handheld
RCM has been used to delineate tumor margins
for lentigo maligna and lentigo maligna melanoma that often exhibit aggressive subclinical
aggression [22–24]. Diagnostic pitfalls include

cases of Spitz, Reed, traumatized, inflamed, or recurrent nevi, which may demonstrate atypical features on RCM imaging [25].

12.2.2 Non-Melanocytic Neoplasms

12.2.2.1 Basal Cell Carcinoma

There are several key RCM features of basal cell carcinoma (BCC) (Table 12.3). Sharply demarcated tumor islands or nodules are often present (Fig. 12.8) and correspond to aggregates of basaloid cells on histopathology [26]. Tumor islands may exhibit palisading or organization of cells with elongated nucleoli around the periphery of the island [27]. Tumor islands may appear bright in pigmented BCC with bright dendritic cells present within the island representing intra-tumoral melanocytes [28]. Tumor islands

Table 12.3 Reflectance confocal microscopy features of basal cell carcinoma

RCM features
– Tumor nodules or islands
– Dark silhouettes and clefting
– Peripheral palisading
– Streaming or polarization
– Cord-like structures at the dermoepidermal junction
– Dilated vessels in the dermis

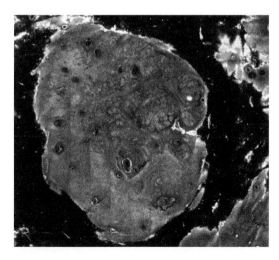

Fig. 12.8 Reflectance confocal microscopy of a basal cell carcinoma with bright and dark tumor lobules, streaming, and palisading

may also appear dark in non-pigmented BCC, with surrounding silhouettes or clefts that likely correspond to mucin on histopathology [27]. Basaloid cells may form cord-like structures at the dermoepidermal junction. Elongated monomorphic keratinocytes that appear to be aligned into the same axis can be visualized at the basal and spinous layers and have been described as streaming or polarization [27, 28]. In the dermis, prominent dilated and tortuous vessel can be visualized, as well as increased bright collagen bundles [28].

RCM has high accuracy in the diagnosis of BCC, with a sensitivity of 82–100% and a specificity of 78–97% [29]. In addition, RCM can help differentiate subtypes of BCC, which may impact management decisions [30]. Superficial BCC is associated with the presence of cords, and nodular BCC is associated with the presence of large tumor nodules and prominent vessels [30]. Infiltrative BCC is difficult to diagnose on RCM due to depth limitations but may be associated with the presence of abundant collagen bundles and the lack of other key features. RCM has also been used to identify biopsy site [31], delineate presurgical tumor margins [32, 33], and monitor response to noninvasive treatment [34, 35].

12.2.2.2 Squamous Cell Carcinoma and Actinic Keratosis

Squamous cell carcinoma (SCC) and actinic keratosis (AK) are characterized by a spectrum of keratinocytic atypia (Table 12.4). RCM features include irregular honeycomb pattern (Fig. 12.9), cellular and nuclear pleiomorphism (Fig. 12.10), and large dyskeratotic cells within the epidermis that may have a targetoid appearance [27]. Hyperkeratosis, parakeratosis, and dilated vessels are also commonly identified. Although it can be difficult to distinguish SCC and AK on RCM, SCC typically displays more severe and widespread keratinocytic and architectural atypia as compared to AK.

RCM has demonstrated a sensitivity of 74–100% and specificity of 78–100% in the diagnosis of SCC [36, 37].

Table 12.4 Reflectance confocal microscopy features of squamous cell carcinoma

RCM features
– Hyperkeratosis
– Parakeratosis
– Irregular honeycomb pattern
– Cellular and nuclear pleiomorphism
– Large apoptotic and dyskeratotic cells
– Dilated vessels in the dermis

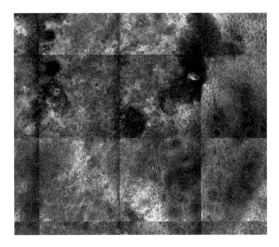

Fig. 12.9 Reflectance confocal microscopy of a squamous cell carcinoma with an irregular honeycomb pattern

12.2.3 Other Applications

12.2.3.1 Infections

RCM can be used to diagnose cutaneous infections in real time (Table 12.5). *Sarcoptes scabiei* infestations can be identified using RCM, and mites and larva appear non-homogenous and highly refractile (Fig. 12.11) [38–40]. *S. scabiei* eggs appear as hyporefractile ovoid structures [39]. RCM can also be used to confirm treatment efficacy with visualization of a dead mite, which appears hyporefractile and with blurred outlines as compared to a live mite [38, 39]. Similarly, *Demodex folliculorum* can be visualized within follicular infundibula [40]. RCM can be used to quantify *Demodex* mites per skin surface area and monitor treatment efficacy over time [41, 42]. Other parasites, such as *Dermanyssus gallinae*, *Ixodes*, *Pediculus humanus*, *Pyemotes ventricosus*, and *Pulex irritans*, have also been detected under RCM [40].

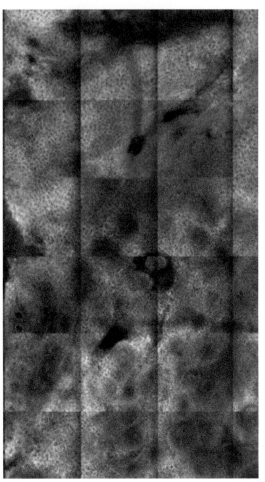

Fig. 12.10 Reflectance confocal microscopy of a squamous cell carcinoma with keratinocytic atypia

Table 12.5 Reflectance confocal microscopy of cutaneous infections

Can be visualized by RCM	Cannot be visualized by RCM
– Parasites	– Viruses[a]
– Fungi	– Bacteria

[a]Cannot visualize viruses on RCM but can visualize viral cytopathological effect on keratinocytes.

RCM can be utilized for rapid diagnosis of dermatophytosis, without the processing time associated with microscopy and culture. Filaments and pseudofilaments can be visualized in the stratum corneum and appear as thin, hyper-reflective, longitudinal structures often with a serpentine shape and occasionally with identi-

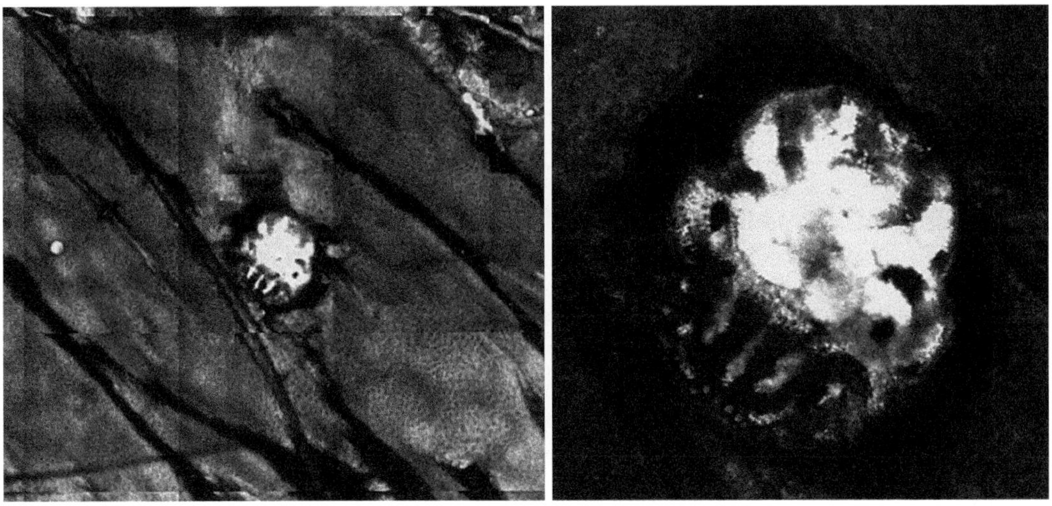

Fig. 12.11 Reflectance confocal microscopy of a pruritic papule shows a *Sarcoptes scabiei* mite

fiable septations [41]. RCM has been used to diagnose skin dermatophytosis, including tinea corporis, tinea manus and pedis, tinea cruris, and tinea incognito, as well as onychomycosis with variable sensitivity and specificity [40, 43, 44].

Individual viruses are too small to identify on RCM; however, viral cytopathological effects on keratinocytes can be visualized. Herpes simplex and herpes zoster are characterized by the presence of dark intraepidermal spaces representing vesicles, acantholytic and dystrophic keratinocytes, multinucleated giant cells, and inflammatory infiltrate [45–47]. *Molluscum contagiosum* is characterized by well-circumscribed cystic areas filled with brightly refractile material that correspond to molluscum inclusion bodies on histology [48]. RCM can provide real-time diagnosis of many inflammatory skin diseases with clinico-confocal correlation.

12.2.3.2 Inflammation

RCM has been used to study inflammatory skin diseases since the late 1990s [40]. There are RCM correlates to the classic histologic features of inflammation. Spongiosis, or intercellular edema, is characterized by larger than normal intercellular spaces between keratinocytes and darker areas in the stratum spinosum [49]. Hyperkeratosis is characterized by a thickened stratum corneum and epidermis, and parakeratosis is character-

ized by refractile nucleated cells in the stratum corneum [49]. Papillomatosis is represented by enlarged and up-located dermal papillae [49]. Inflammatory cells are hyper-refractile on RCM imaging and appear as small bright cells. Dilated vessels are characterized by large, dark round, or canalicular structures.

RCM can be used to diagnose inflammatory skin diseases with the identification of these features (Table 12.6). Spongiotic dermatitis is characterized by irregular honeycomb pat-

Table 12.6 Inflammatory patterns on reflectance confocal microscopy

Inflammatory pattern	RCM features
Spongiotic	– Irregular honeycomb pattern – Spongiosis – Epidermal inflammatory infiltrate – Perivascular inflammatory infiltrate – Dilated vessels
Psoriasiform	– Hyperkeratosis – Papillomatosis – Epidermal inflammatory infiltrates (neutrophilic lakes) – Dilated vessels
Interface	– Dermoepidermal junction obscuration – Inflammatory infiltrate at the dermoepidermal junction

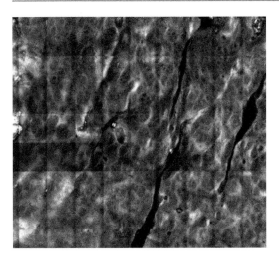

Fig. 12.12 Reflectance confocal microscopy of a psoriatic plaque shows marked papillomatosis and dilated vessels

tern, spongiosis, epidermal and perivascular inflammatory infiltrate, and dilated vessels [49, 50]. Psoriasiform dermatitis is characterized by hyperkeratosis, papillomatosis, epidermal inflammatory infiltrates corresponding to neutrophilic lakes, and dilated vessels (Fig. 12.12) [49, 50]. Interface dermatitis is characterized by dermoepidermal junction obscuration and inflammatory infiltrate at the dermoepidermal junction [49, 50]. There is a wide range of values reported for disease-specific sensitivity and specificity, and clinico-confocal correlation is necessary [40]. RCM can also be used to monitor inflammatory skin disease over time.

12.2.3.3 Burns and Wound Healing

Recent studies have explored RCM imaging of burn [51, 52] and other wounds [53–57] to track and predict healing.

12.3 Advantages and Disadvantages

While skin biopsy and traditional histopathology remain the gold standard for the diagnosis of skin disease, RCM affords many benefits for patients and providers. RCM is noninvasive and painless, capable of imaging in vivo live skin, and time efficient, with imaging of a single lesion completed in 10–15 min. RCM generates images with cellular-level resolution, and RCM diagnosis has consistently demonstrated high sensitivity and specificity when compared to histopathology [58, 59]. Thus, the use of RCM can spare patients unnecessary biopsies and avoid the risk for bleeding, surgical site infections, and scarring. These benefits appeal to both patients and providers, especially with lesions in cosmetically sensitive areas such as the face. Furthermore, dermatologists and dermatopathologists are reimbursed for image acquisition and interpretation [3].

However, there are several limitations of RCM. Images are generated in grayscale, which can be more challenging to interpret as compared to colored hematoxylin and eosin dyes. RCM has a maximum depth of 200–300 μm varying with body site, limiting evaluation of pathology in the deep dermis [7]. In addition, it can be challenging to evaluate certain lesions, such as ulcerated lesions and burn wounds, as imaging requires direct contact with the scope and the lesion. There can also be poor diagnostic specificity with certain confocal features. Bright dendritic cells may represent atypical melanocytes but may also represent Langerhans cells [60]. It can also be challenging to differentiate vellus hair follicles and eccrine ducts from the dark tumor nodules of basal cell carcinoma [61]. Furthermore, although confocal morphology is similar to that of traditional histopathology, the accurate interpretation of grayscale en face images requires considerable training and practice [20, 61].

12.4 Conclusion

Reflectance confocal microscopy is a noninvasive imaging modality that has a wide range of applications, encompassing the diagnosis and treatment monitoring of cutaneous neoplasms and inflammatory skin disease.

References

1. Minsky M. Memoir on inventing the confocal scanning microscope. Scanning. 1988;10:128–38.
2. Rajadhyaksha M, González S, Zavislan JM, Anderson RR, Webb RH. In vivo confocal scanning laser microscopy of human skin II: advances in instrumentation and comparison with histology. J Invest Dermatol. 1999;113(3):293–303.
3. Current Procedural Terminology, Professional Edition. Chicago IL: American Medical Association; 2016. The preliminary physician fee schedule for 2017 is available at https://www.cms.gov/Medicare/Medicare-Fee-for-Service-Payment/PhysicianFeeSched/PFS-Federal-Regulation-Notices-Items/CMS-1654-P.html.
4. Yamashita T, Kuwahara T, González S, Takahashi M. Non-invasive visualization of melanin and melanocytes by reflectance-mode confocal microscopy. J Invest Dermatol. 2005;124(1):235–40.
5. Rajadhyaksha M, Grossman M, Esterowitz D, Webb HR, Anderson RR. In vivo confocal scanning laser microscopy of human skin: melanin provides strong contrast. J Invest Dermatol. 1995;104(6):946–52.
6. Rao BK, Pellacani G. Atlas of confocal microscopy in dermatology: clinical, confocal, and histological images. New York: NIDIskin LLC; 2013.
7. Scope A, et al. In vivo reflectance confocal microscopy imaging of melanocytic skin lesions: consensus terminology glossary and illustrative images. J Am Acad Dermatol. 2007;57(4):644–58.
8. Pellacani G, et al. The impact of in vivo reflectance confocal microscopy for the diagnostic accuracy of melanoma and equivocal melanocytic lesions. J Invest Dermatol. 2007;127(12):2759–65.
9. Segura S, Puig S, Carrera C, Palou J, Malvehy J. Development of a two-step method for the diagnosis of melanoma by reflectance confocal microscopy. J Am Acad Dermatol. 2009;61(2):216–29.
10. Guitera P, et al. In vivo confocal microscopy for diagnosis of melanoma and basal cell carcinoma using a two-step method: analysis of 710 consecutive clinically equivocal cases. J Invest Dermatol. 2012;132(10):2386–94.
11. Pellacani G, et al. In vivo confocal microscopy for detection and grading of dysplastic nevi: a pilot study. J Am Acad Dermatol. 2012;66(3):e109–21.
12. Pellacani G, et al. Towards an in vivo morphologic classification of melanocytic nevi. J Eur Acad Dermatol Venereol. 2014;28(7):864–72.
13. Guitera P, Pellacani G, Crotty KA, Scolyer RA, Li LX, Bassoli S, et al. The impact of in vivo reflectance confocal microscopy on the diagnostic accuracy of lentigo maligna and equivocal pigmented and non-pigmented macules of the face. J Invest Dermatol. 2010;130(8):2080–91.
14. Gerger A, Hofmann-Wellenhof R, Langsenlehner U, et al. *In vivo* confocal laser scanning microscopy of melanocytic skin tumours: diagnostic applicability using unselected tumour images. Br J Dermatol. 2008;158(2):329–33.
15. Stevenson AD, Mickan S, Mallett S, Ayya M. Systematic review of diagnostic accuracy of reflectance confocal microscopy for melanoma diagnosis in patients with clinically equivocal skin lesions. Dermatol Pract Concept. 2013;3(4):19–27.
16. Alarcon I, Carrera C, Palou J, Alos L, Malvehy J, Puig S. Impact of in vivo reflectance confocal microscopy on the number needed to treat melanoma in doubtful lesions. Br J Dermatol. 2014;170(4):802–8.
17. Lovatto L, Carrera C, Salerni G, Alós L, Malvehy J, Puig S. In vivo reflectance confocal microscopy of equivocal melanocytic lesions detected by digital dermoscopy follow-up. J Eur Acad Dermatol Venereol. 2015;29(10):1918–25.
18. Guitera P, et al. In vivo reflectance confocal microscopy enhances secondary evaluation of melanocytic lesions. J Invest Dermatol. 2009;129(1):131–8.
19. Xiong YQ, et al. Comparison of dermoscopy and reflectance confocal microscopy for the diagnosis of malignant skin tumours: a meta-analysis. J Cancer Res Clin Oncol. 2017;143(9):1627–35.
20. Rao BK, Mateus R, Wassef C, Pellacani G. In vivo confocal microscopy in clinical practice: comparison of bedside diagnostic accuracy of a trained physician and distant diagnosis of an expert reader. J Am Acad Dermatol. 2013;69(6):e295–300.
21. Guitera P, et al. Dermoscopy and in vivo confocal microscopy are complementary techniques for diagnosis of difficult amelanotic and light-coloured skin lesions. Br J Dermatol. 2016;175(6):1311–9.
22. Pellacani G, et al. The smart approach: feasibility of lentigo maligna superficial margin assessment with hand-held reflectance confocal microscopy technology. J Eur Acad Dermatol Venereol. 2018;32(10):1687–94.
23. Yélamos O, et al. Correlation of handheld reflectance confocal microscopy with radial video mosaicing for margin mapping of lentigo maligna and lentigo maligna melanoma. JAMA Dermatol. 2017;153(12):1278–84.
24. Champin J, et al. In vivo reflectance confocal microscopy to optimize the spaghetti technique for defining surgical margins of lentigo maligna. Dermatol Surg. 2014;40(3):247–56.
25. Waddell A, Star P, Guitera P. Advances in the use of reflectance confocal microscopy in melanoma. Melanoma Manag. 2018;5(1):MMT04.
26. González S, Tannous Z. Real-time, in vivo confocal reflectance microscopy of basal cell carcinoma. J Am Acad Dermatol. 2002;47(6):869–74.
27. Navarrete-Dechent C, et al. Reflectance confocal microscopy terminology glossary for nonmelanocytic skin lesions: a systematic review. J Am Acad Dermatol. 2019;80:1414–27.
28. Ahlgrimm-Siess V, et al. Confocal microscopy in skin cancer. Curr Dermatol Rep. 2018;7(2):105–18.
29. Kadouch DJ, et al. In vivo confocal microscopy of basal cell carcinoma: a systematic review of

diagnostic accuracy. J Eur Acad Dermatol Venereol. 2015;29(10):1890–7.

30. Longo C, et al. Classifying distinct basal cell carcinoma subtype by means of dermatoscopy and reflectance confocal microscopy. J Am Acad Dermatol. 2014;71(4):716–724.e1.

31. Navarrete-Dechent C, Mori S, Cordova M, Nehal KS. Reflectance confocal microscopy as a novel tool for presurgical identification of basal cell carcinoma biopsy site. J Am Acad Dermatol. 2019;80(1):e7–8.

32. Pan ZY, Lin JR, Cheng TT, Wu JQ, Wu WY. In vivo reflectance confocal microscopy of Basal cell carcinoma: feasibility of preoperative mapping of cancer margins. Dermatol Surg. 2012;38(12):1945–50.

33. Venturini M, Gualdi G, Zanca A, Lorenzi L, Pellacani G, Calzavara-Pinton PG. A new approach for presurgical margin assessment by reflectance confocal microscopy of basal cell carcinoma. Br J Dermatol. 2016;174:380–5.

34. Sierra H, Yélamos O, Cordova M, Chen CJ, Rajadhyaksha M. Reflectance confocal microscopy-guided laser ablation of basal cell carcinomas: initial clinical experience. J Biomed Opt. 2017;22:1–13.

35. Maier T, Kulichova D, Ruzicka T, Berking C. Noninvasive monitoring of basal cell carcinomas treated with systemic hedgehog inhibitors: pseudocysts as a sign of tumor regression. J Am Acad Dermatol. 2014;71(4):725–30.

36. Dinnes J, et al. Reflectance confocal microscopy for diagnosing keratinocyte skin cancers in adults. Cochrane Database Syst Rev. 2018;12:CD013191.

37. Nguyen KP, Peppelman M, Hoogedoorn L, Van Erp PE, Gerritsen MP. The current role of in vivo reflectance confocal microscopy within the continuum of actinic keratosis and squamous cell carcinoma: a systematic review. Eur J Dermatol. 2016;26(6):549–65.

38. Francisco G, et al. No wonder it itches: quick bedside visualization of a scabies infestation using reflectance confocal microscopy. J Cutan Pathol. 2018;45(12):877–9.

39. Cinotti E, Perrot J-L, Labeille B, Cambazard F. On the feasibility of confocal microscopy for the diagnosis of scabies. Ann Dermatol Venereol. 2013;140:215–6.

40. Hoogedoorn L, Peppelman M, van de Kerkhof PC, van Erp PE, Gerritsen MJ. The value of in vivo reflectance confocal microscopy in the diagnosis and monitoring of inflammatory and infectious skin diseases: a systematic review. Br J Dermatol. 2015;172(5):1222–48.

41. Cinotti E, Perrot JL, Labeille B, Cambazard F. Reflectance confocal microscopy for cutaneous infections and infestations. J Eur Acad Dermatol Venereol. 2016;30(5):754–63.

42. Ruini C, Sattler E, Hartmann D, Reinholz M, Ruzicka T, von Braunmühl T. Monitoring structural changes in Demodex mites under topical Ivermectin in rosacea by means of reflectance confocal microscopy: a case series. J Eur Acad Dermatol Venereol. 2017;31(6):e299–301.

43. Pharaon M, Gari-Toussaint M, Khemis A, et al. Diagnosis and treatment monitoring of toenail onychomycosis by reflectance confocal microscopy: prospective cohort study in 58 patients. J Am Acad Dermatol. 2014;71:56–61.

44. Hui D, Xue-cheng S, Ai-e X. Evaluation of reflectance confocal microscopy in dermatophytosis. Mycoses. 2013;56:130–3.

45. Lacarrubba F, Verzì AE, Pippione M, Micali G. Reflectance confocal microscopy in the diagnosis of vesicobullous disorders: case series with pathologic and cytologic correlation and literature review. Skin Res Technol. 2016;22(4):479–86.

46. Debarbieux S, Depaepe L, Poulalhon N, Dalle S, Balme B, Thomas L. Reflectance confocal microscopy characteristics of eight cases of pustular eruptions and histopathological correlations. Skin Res Technol. 2013;19(1):e444–52.

47. Goldgeier M, Alessi C, Muhlbauer JE. Immediate noninvasive diagnosis of herpesvirus by confocal scanning laser microscopy. J Am Acad Dermatol. 2002;46(5):783–5.

48. Scope A, Benvenuto-Andrade C, Gill M, Ardigo M, Gonzalez S, Marghoob AA. Reflectance confocal microscopy of molluscum contagiosum. Arch Dermatol. 2008;144:34.

49. Ardigo M, Longo C, Gonzalez S. International Confocal Working Group Inflammatory Skin Diseases Project. Multicentre study on inflammatory skin diseases from The International Confocal Working Group: specific confocal microscopy features and an algorithmic method of diagnosis. Br J Dermatol. 2016;175(2):364–74.

50. Ardigo M, Agozzino M, Franceschini C, Lacarrubba F. Reflectance confocal microscopy algorithms for inflammatory and hair diseases. Dermatol Clin. 2016;34(4):487–96.

51. Iftimia N, et al. Combined reflectance confocal microscopy/optical coherence tomography imaging for skin burn assessment. Biomed Opt Express. 2013;4(5):680–95.

52. Altintas AA, et al. To heal or not to heal: predictive value of in vivo reflectance-mode confocal microscopy in assessing healing course of human burn wounds. J Burn Care Res. 2009;30(6):1007–12.

53. Srivastava R, Reilly C, Francisco GM, Bhatti H, Rao BK. Life of a wound: serial documentation of wound healing after shave removal using reflectance confocal microscopy. J Drugs Dermatol. 2019;18(5):217–9.

54. Cameli N, Mariano M, Serio M, Ardigò M. Preliminary comparison of fractional laser with fractional laser plus radiofrequency for the treatment of acne scars and photoaging. Dermatol Surg. 2014;40(5):553–61.

55. Stumpp OF, Bedi VP, Wyatt D, Lac D, et al. In vivo confocal imaging of epidermal cell migration and dermal changes post nonablative fractional resurfacing: study of the wound healing process with corroborated histopathologic evidence. J Biomed Opt. 2009;14(2):024018.

56. Terhorst D, Maltusch A, Stockfleth E, Lange-Asschenfeldt S, et al. Reflectance confocal microscopy

for the evaluation of acute epidermal wound healing. Wound Repair Regen. 2011;19(6):671–9.

57. Lange-Asschenfeldt S, Bob A, Terhorst D, Ulrich M, et al. Applicability of confocal laser scanning microscopy for evaluation and monitoring of cutaneous wound healing. J Biomed Opt. 2012;17(7):076016.

58. Rajadhyaksha M, Marghoob A, Rossi A, Halpern AC, Nehal KS. Reflectance confocal microscopy of skin in vivo: from bench to bedside. Lasers Surg Med. 2017;49(1):7–19.

59. Rao BK, John AM, Francisco G, Haroon A. Diagnostic accuracy of reflectance confocal microscopy skin. Arch Pathol Lab Med. 2019;143:326–9.

60. Hashemi P, et al. Langerhans cells and melanocytes share similar morphologic features under in vivo reflectance confocal microscopy: a challenge for melanoma diagnosis. J Am Acad Dermatol. 2012;66(3):452–62. https://doi.org/10.1016/j.jaad.2011.02.033.

61. Jain M, Pulijal SV, Rajadhyaksha M, Halpern AC, Gonzalez S. Evaluation of bedside diagnostic accuracy, learning curve, and challenges for a novice reflectance confocal microscopy reader for skin cancer detection in vivo. JAMA Dermatol. 2018;154(8):962–5.